AN INTRODUCTION TO
VOICE PATHOLOGY

AN INTRODUCTION TO VOICE PATHOLOGY

Functional and Organic

By

P. H. DAMSTÉ, M.D.
Department of Phoniatry
University of Utrecht
Medical School
Utrecht, Netherlands

and

J. W. LERMAN, Ph.D.
Department of Speech
University of Connecticut
Storrs, Connecticut

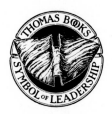

CHARLES C THOMAS · PUBLISHER
Springfield · Illinois · U.S.A.

Published and Distributed Throughout the World by
CHARLES C THOMAS • PUBLISHER
Bannerstone House
301-327 East Lawrence Avenue, Springfield, Illinois, U.S.A.

© 1975, by CHARLES C THOMAS • PUBLISHER
ISBN 0-398-03289-0
Library of Congress Catalog Card Number: 74-20858

With THOMAS BOOKS *careful attention is given to all details of manufacturing and design. It is the Publisher's desire to present books that are satisfactory as to their physical qualities and artistic possibilities and appropriate for their particular use.* THOMAS BOOKS *will be true to those laws of quality that assure a good name and good will.*

Printed in the United States of America
W-2

Library of Congress Cataloging in Publication Data

Damsté, Pieter Helbert.
    An introduction to voice pathology, functional and organic.

    Bibliography: p.
    Includes index.
    1. Speech, Disorders of. I. Lerman, Jay William, 1929-   joint author.   II. Title. [DNLM: 1. Speech disorders. 2. Voice. WV500 D166i]
RC423.D2   616.8'55   74-20858
ISBN 0-398-03289-0

FOREWORD

THIS BOOK IS designed as an introductory text for speech clinicians at all levels of training and for otorhinolaryngologists, whether in residence or practice. It is intended not to answer, or even raise, all the questions in the area of voice pathology, but rather to interest and entice the reader to seek further. Hence, the simplistic treatment of often complex content has been a purposeful approach in this book.

In attempting to present a total, yet compact, view of voice pathology for the speech clinician and the medical profession, the book is not consistent in style throughout; some subjects are discussed in a rather elementary manner, while more complicated areas are treated with greater sophistication. Further, to accomplish clarity and readability without oversimplification, some detailed information had to be omitted.

Some of the issues discussed in this text may appear to be controversial, in that we have stressed many concepts which are the backbone of clinical practice even if experimental proof has not yet been brought forward. There is a "wide chasm between science in the laboratory and practice in the field," and the tone of this book then, in part, connotes that clinical experience cannot, and need not, always wait for experimental evidence in order to be accorded serious potential credibility.

In the final analysis then, the primary purpose of the book is to introduce the speech clinician and others to some of the basic concepts of voice pathology as we view them. This book is of interest to the researcher only insofar as he may want to orient himself to various aspects of voice disorders, and as it may serve as an incentive for selection of an area for research.

P.H.D.
J.W.L.

CONTENTS

AN INTRODUCTION TO
VOICE PATHOLOGY

Chapter 1

THE FUNCTIONING LARYNX

L ANGUAGE AND THE process of verbal abstraction is particular to man; but voice, or the ability to produce sound, is common to both man and animals. Voice is a product of nature and has existed in man's repertoire much longer than language, which is a product of culture. We know that most animals are able to make sound or noises which have distinct meaning to other members of their group. By means of a system of warning cries young crows learn from older ones what potential dangers and enemies they must heed. Singing birds mark the boundaries of their territories and ward off intruders with repeated monologues (Kainz, 1961; Lorenz, 1962).

Many species, however, make very little use of the phonatory possibilities of their sound-producing mechanism. The salamander, for instance, has a simple sphincter reinforced by two pieces of cartilage which closes off the trachea from the pharynx. Although he can make some noises with it, he communicates solely by gesture. Primates, who are most closely related to man, have all the necessary vocal apparatus used in the production of speech, but rely mostly on a gesture language. On the basis of more contemporary literature we can only state that the primates have less developed abstracting functions of the brain and have not developed the stage of verbal language which is a vehicle for messages of intellectual content. Nonetheless, the animal world provides sufficient examples of sounds as a communication network in the absence of the complicated symbols of human language.

The larynx developed initially as a primitive sphincter which could close off the airway during the act of swallowing. At the present time the functional possibilities of the larynx have increased considerably due to the differentiation of the cartilage structure and the extraordinary grouping of the muscle bundles derived from the original sphincter. We must realize that the human larynx is better equipped than that of any other species for the "language" of voice.

THE STRUCTURE OF THE LARYNX

The great variability of the human voice regarding pitch and quality is basically due to (1) the movement of the cricothyroid articulation; (2) the arytenoids (each in their position in the center of four muscles, and gliding and rocking on a rather large articulating surface of the cricoid, acting as a lever or pulley to change the direction of forces); and (3) the connective tissue membrane, conus elasticus, that is draped between the upper rim of the cricoid and a line between the vocal process of the arytenoid and the anterior commissure of the thyroid.

A thorough understanding of the physiological processes involved in voice production is necessary. The present chapter is not intended to be a detailed analysis of the anatomy and physiology of the sound-producing mechanism, but a concise survey of the laryngeal structures. The information is presented simply and basically to facilitate understanding of other concepts to be discussed later. Some excellent books are recommended for detailed discussion of the anatomy and physiology of the sound-producing mechanism (Kaplan, 1960; Judson and Weaver, 1965; Zemlin, 1968, and others).

Cartilages of the Larynx

The larynx consists of nine cartilages. These are the thyroid, cricoid, and epiglottis (all unpaired); and the paired arytenoids, corniculates, and cuneiforms. Only the thyroid, cricoid, and arytenoid cartilages will be discussed.

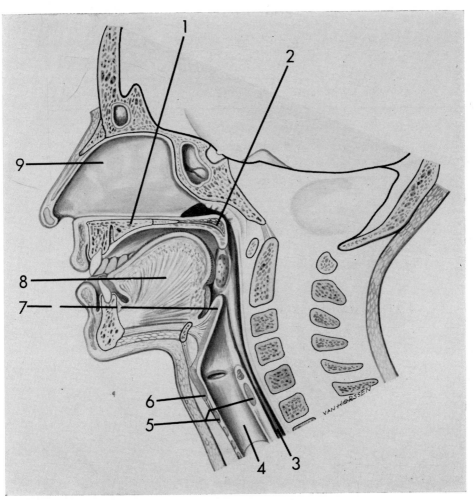

Figure 1. Sagittal section of head and neck showing relationships of nasal, oral, and pharyngeal cavities. (1) hard palate, (2) soft palate, (3) esophagus, (4) trachea, (5) cricoid cartilage, (6) thyroid cartilage, (7) epiglottis, (8) tongue, (9) nasal septum. "From: De pathologische stembandfunctie Stafleu, Leiden Neth."

Thyroid Cartilage

This is the most prominent cartilage of the laryngeal structure. It is made up of two parts called the laminae. At the anterior point of fusion of these two plates the thyroid is seen as a blunt projection commonly called the "Adam's Apple" (laryngeal prominence). At the posterior section of each of these plates can be seen superior and inferior horns. This backward deviation gives the cartilage an open V-shape, with the superior horn directed upward and attached to the hyoid bone by ligaments. The inferior horn inclines downward to articulate with the cricoid cartilage. Attached at the internal surface of the thyroid notch (the point at which the laminae are fused) are ligaments and muscles important in the production of sound.

Cricoid Cartilage

This is also an unpaired cartilage lying just below the thyroid cartilage and just above the tracheal cartilages. Its shape has often been compared to a signet ring, with the front and sides of the cartilage forming a narrow arch, and the posterior portion or laminae being a vertical plate somewhat hexagonal in shape. The upper border of this posterior plate is shaped so as to provide surfaces of articulation for the arytenoid cartilages.

Arytenoid Cartilages

These two pyramid-shaped cartilages are located atop the laminae of the cricoid cartilage. Each of these has a base and an apex. The base is concave, which allows it to rest on the corresponding convex portion of the cricoid cartilage. At the base of this cartilage are the vocal process and the muscular process. The muscular process is a posteriolateral projection (that is, directed backwards and sidewards) and gives attachment or provides insertion for muscles. The vocal process is directed forward and is so called because of the fold (vocal) attached to it.

Laryngeal Joints

Not only do the joints help to unite the laryngeal cartilages, but they assist in the positioning and tensing of the vocal folds. Two of the joints in the larynx are the cricoarytenoid and the cricothyroid.

The Cricoarytenoid Joint

This is formed by the aforementioned concavity in the underside of the base of the arytenoid cartilage and the corresponding convex surface on the top of the laminae of the cricoid cartilage. It is a synovial-type joint, enclosed by a fibrous capsular ligament. Investigation by Sonesson (1959) has revealed that the point of articulation on the laminae of the cricoid is not in a horizontal position but rather in an oblique position, which then allows the pivotal rotation of the joint to be on an oblique course. Sonesson (1968) further states that this joint permits the arytenoid cartilage two types of movement: rotation and translation (gliding movement).

> At the rotation, the vocal process is either raised and at the same time carried laterally, or is lowered, and at the same time carried inwards toward the midline through the larynx. At the translation movement, the arytenoid cartilage is displaced along the axis of rotation, whether in direction obliquely forward and downward or obliquely. These oblique rotation movements mean that the vocal folds might change their position in space, not only laterally and medially, but also in a superior and inferior direction.

The Cricothyroid Joint

This joint is formed by the inferior horn of the thyroid cartilage articulating with the small oval articular facets on the outside of the arch of the cricoid cartilage. This point of articulation allows for the rotation of the cricoid cartilage. If the arch of the cricoid is rotated or tilted upward, the lamina is rotated backward and downward, resulting in a lengthening of the vocal folds. When the cricoid arch is lowered, it is moved away from the thyroid cartilage and the vocal folds are thus shortened. Therefore, although the thyroid cartilage itself does not perform any rotation movements, the rotational movements allowed by this joint is one of several factors related to pitch change in the human voice.

Ardran and Kemp (1967) discuss in greater detail the movements of the arytenoid and cricoid cartilages and their relationships to changes in vocal fold length. Hollien (1962) and Hollien and Curtis (1960, 1962) have done some extremely interesting measurements of vocal fold thickness and length. Their research indicates that one of the more important factors relating to vocal pitch and pitch change is that of mass or thickness of the vocal folds and that a relationship does exist between vocal fold tilt and increase in vocal pitch.

Laryngeal Membranes

There are many membranes and ligaments connecting the cartilages of the larynx, but our purposes would be best served in discussing only two: the aryepiglottic folds and the conus elasticus.

The Aryepiglottic Folds

These paired folds form the opening into the larynx. The muscle fibers flow between the arytenoid cartilages and the epiglottis on the lateral sides. Some individuals feel that the aryepiglottic folds are sphincter-like in action and aid in the active closure of the larynx by folding together when the larynx is elevated to meet the base of the tongue. It is possible that this narrowing of the entrance is more of a passive event resulting from the pharyngeal constriction and elevation of the larynx. Cleary (1954) has written a very definitive description of these folds.

The Conus Elasticus

The conus elasticus, indicated aptly by Merkel (1863) as the voice membrane, covers the muscles of the vocal fold, the internal and external thyroarytenoid muscles. It also helps connect the cricoid, thyroid, and arytenoid cartilages. Single fibers of the muscles of the vocal fold insert into the voice membrane. Because of this connection with the underlying muscles and the upper free rim of the voice membrane (1) the vocal ligament can be adjusted in a lower and higher position, and (2) the voice membrane can be flaccid and supple, or stretched and stiff.

Muscles of the Larynx

These have always been referred to as the intrinsic and extrinsic musculature. The extrinsic group connects the larynx with those parts of the skeleton outside of the laryngeal area, while the intrinsic group is concerned with the laryngeal cartilages themselves. Sonesson (1968) proposes a better designation

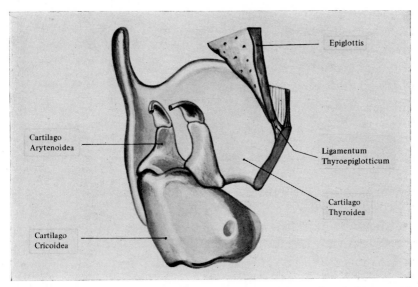

Figure 2. The voice membranes run from the inner side of the cricoid to the medial side of the vocal folds. The free ending upper rims are the vocal ligaments.

for the intrinsic musculature, the "proper laryngeal muscles," and for the extrinsic group, "supra- and infrahyoidal muscles."

The proper laryngeal muscles consist of those muscles used for adduction (closing of the glottis) and the lone abductor (opening of the glottis), the paired posterior cricoarytenoid muscles.

The lateral cricoarytenoid muscles, which originate at the arch of the cricoid and insert in the front part of the muscular processes of the arytenoid, are situated outside the external and internal thyro-arytenoid, or vocalis muscles, and can be viewed as the outer part of the original sphincter. They rotate the arytenoids in such a fashion that the vocal processes move medially (in a direction approaching each other) wherein the glottis closes without shortening, as would be the case if the muscles acted as a sphincter. The contracting lateral cricoarytenoid makes the arytenoid cartilage tilt over the rim of the cricoid cartilage so that the vocal process points downward; in adducted position, during phonation, the vocal folds are lower (more caudal) than in the abducted position. Thus, on adduction the conus elasticus, the connective tissue on the medial sides of the folds, is relaxed. We, therefore, have a relaxed or flaccid, supple inner part of the glottal sphincter in a firmly contracted outer part.

The interarytenoid muscle, which is situated more cranially, originates from the lateral margin and muscular process of one arytenoid cartilage crossing over in a horizontal position to the lateral edge of the other arytenoid cartilage. Activity in this muscle closes the posterior cartilaginous part of the glottis.

The thyroarytenoid or vocalis muscle, which consists of several parts, originates chiefly from the angle of the thyroid cartilage and extends to the vocal process of the arytenoid cartilage. With the held of this muscle the elasticity or firmness of the vocal fold is adjusted.

The cricothyroid muscle is a muscle of two parts, originating in the lateral arch of the cricoid cartilage and inserting into the thyroid cartilage. Together with the suspension system of the larynx this muscle determines the length of the vocal folds. It tilts the posterior cricoid plate backwards; and as a result, the arytenoid cartilages, connected to the cricoid cartilage, are also tilted. This action increases the distance between the anterior insertion of the vocal folds, at the angle of the thyroid, and the posterior insertion on the vocal process of the arytenoid cartilages, thus stretching the vocal ligaments.

The extrinsic, or supra- and infrahyoidal muscles, as well as the pharyngeal musculature support the laryngeal structure, fixing it in various positions. They are sometimes referred to as the "strap" muscles. They both elevate (suprahyoid) and depress (infrahyoid) the larynx, and thereby exert considerable influence on sound production.

Those muscles which aid in raising the laryngeal structure via the hyoid bone are the stylohyoid, genio-hyoid, hyoglossus, digastricus, and others. These make up the suprahyoid musculature. Faaborg-Andersen and Sonninen (1959) have shown that as pitch increases there is an increase in the levator action of these muscles (as well as an increase in activity of those muscles which pull the larynx down). This combination of activity causes a forward and very slight upward movement of the larynx during phonation.

The depressors of infrahyoid muscles are the thyrohyoid, sternothyroid, and sternohyoid. Sonninen (1956) reported that the sternothyroid muscles will move the entire laryngeal structure down and, dependent upon other factors such as head and neck position and action of other proper laryngeal musculature, the vocal folds will be shortened or lengthened.

Of the muscles of the pharynx, the one that may be the most closely related to sound generation is the cricopharyngeus. This band of muscle fibers is part of the inferior constrictor muscle; it originates on the lateral aspects of the cricoid cartilage and inserts into a tendinous strip in the medial portion of the posterior pharyngeal wall. Zenker and Zenker (1960) have shown that because of its point of insertion the cricopharyngeus muscle is able to elevate the posterior plate of the cricoid cartilage, hence offsetting the cricothyroid muscle and shortening the folds. Sonninen (1956) states that such an action is only possible when the position of the larynx is low. If the larynx is raised cranially, it is not possible for the cricopharyngeus to shorten the folds.

This short summary of muscle function can serve as a basis for understanding the mechanism by which frequency and the form of the vocal fold vibrations are controlled. Faaborg-Andersen and Sonninen (1959), Faaborg-Andersen and Vennard (1964), and Zenker and Zenker (1960) have pursued further the functioning of the suspension system and its effect on changes in size and shape of the vocal folds.

THE LARYNX IN FUNCTION

Before proceeding with the mechanism of phonation, it is well to remember that the larynx has some more vital functions other than that of a voice organ.

Protection of the Lower Airway

The larynx can be closed on three levels: (1) the vocal folds,

(2) the ventricular folds, and (3) the laryngeal entrance (the aryepiglottic folds). This aspect of laryngeal function is most clearly manifested in the act of *swallowing*. In swallowing one is able to observe that the larynx, together with the hyoid bone, is displaced upward. In yawning, on the contrary, the tongue-hyoid-larynx complex is moved in a caudal direction. This freedom of movement is due to the fact that the hyoid and larynx are suspended in a system of long muscles. The only exception is the cricopharyngeal muscle which attaches the larynx to the vertebral column. This is a short muscle (previously described) that in itself is somewhat moveable vis-á-vis to the vertebral column.

The swallowing reflex allows food on its way to the esophagus to have a level crossing with the airway. The airway is closed momentarily by a strong cranial movement of the larynx which meets the base of the tongue as it is moved backwards. The epiglottis, which is in between, protects the airway in such a way that food is channeled into the piriform sinuses on both sides. The piriform sinus acts as a guide tract from the hypopharynx to the mouth of the esophagus. At that moment the entrance of the larynx is further protected when the aryepiglottic folds, which are reinforced with small pieces of cartilage, are pushed together. They fill the spaces left on both sides when the arytenoids position themselves against the tuberculum epiglottis. The small quantity that may have intruded in the laryngeal vestibule is squeezed back during the next phase of swallowing by a simultaneous contraction of the entire laryngeal sphincter at the moment that the mouth of the esophagus opens. It is necessary that the muscle contractions be well-coordinated; otherwise an accident commonly known as "going down the wrong pipe" may occur. The swallowing act has been explored in detail by Ardran and Kemp (1956), Bosma (1957) and Bosma, Sheets, and Shelton (1960).

When some matter does intrude into the larynx, the *coughing reflex* comes into action. It is triggered by the stimulation of the epithelium of the larynx and the lower airway. The reflectory constriction of the larynx is followed by a sudden expiration which has an explosive character. The vocal folds and the ventricular and aryepiglottic folds are shaken vehemently by the turbulent airstream. The effect is that all the foreign bodies and some phlegm are thrown off. They will be ejected into the outside air via the oral cavity and/or they will be thrown into the walls of the pharynx and oral cavity and may be removed by swallowing.

A particularly threatening situation for the airway is the *vomiting reflex.* The contents of an overloaded, irritated stomach then has to pass the aforementioned level of crossing in a reverse direction. This passing takes place in an unexpected and involuntary moment with the possibility that some of this matter may find its way into the trachea. However, when the vomiting reflex occurs, the antiperistaltic constriction of the stomach walls elicits a strong closure of all three levels of the laryngeal sphincter before the reflex has arrived at the wall of the pharynx. Subsequently the pharynx is maximally constricted and the velum is elevated so that the undesired ingesta are ejected via the oral cavity.

PHONATION

People who have had laryngectomies have a way of speaking in which the epithelium of the mouth of the esophagus is brought into vibration: esophageal speech. This clearly proves that a simple sphincter, covered with epithelium, is capable of producing a voice that is adequate for speech. This substitute voice organ has been called a pseudoglottis or neoglottis. It has also been suggested that we consider the term paleoglottis; the laryngectomized has regressed to a mechanism of voice production that existed prior to the mesozoicum. Even amphibians are better equipped for phonation, although they make less practical use of it. (More about the problem of laryngectomy and the laryngectomized will be found in Chapter 8.)

Concerning vocal fold vibration, the "neurochronaxic" theory evolved by Husson (1950, 1960) suggests that vibrations of the vocal folds are caused by active contractions of the vocalis muscles at the rate of the impulses' arriving via the recurrent laryngeal nerves. The frequency of vibration of the folds thus would depend upon the rate of impulses activating the proper laryngeal muscles with subglottic air pressure facilitating greater amplitude of the opening phase. However, all reliable experimental evidence (Rubin, 1960; van den Berg, 1958; and Dedo and Dunker, 1967) relating to this theoretical concept tends to negate it.

The classic myoelastic-aerodynamic theory, which is the most generally accepted, states that vocal folds are tensed and placed in position by the action of the laryngeal muscles, then set into vibration by subglottic air pressure. The vocal folds themselves are passive, but when they are in an adducted position subglottal (below the level of the vocal folds) air pressure builds up until it overcomes the resistance of the vocal folds. When a puff of air passes, there is a reduction in subglottal air presusre, and the vocal folds return to their closed position through their own elasticity and the suction effect of the airflow (Bernoulli effect). This process is repeated until the cords are separated. The frequency of vibration of the folds is dependent upon, among other things, the degree of airflow through the glottis. This in turn depends upon the closure of the glottis and the length, shape, and elasticity (suppleness and firmness) of the vocal folds.

> During the production of sound, the vocal folds are in the adducted position. In this position they vibrate, alternately opening and closing the glottis for very short periods. . . .
>
> The open and closed period is called the vibratory cycle. Because of the rapid vibratory movements of the vocal folds, the duration cycle is very short: in the male speech only 1/125 second and in the female half that time . . .
>
> The vibratory movements of the vocal folds are rather complex especially in low frequencies. Large surfaces of the vocal folds are there in contact with each other during the closure period . . . When the opening is to occur the separation of the vocal folds does not occur in one movement, but it starts from underneath, the opening progressing upwards, and not until the upper parts have separated does the glottis open. This means that the glottis is actually closed during about one third of the phonation time, at least at low . . . frequencies (Sonesson, 1968).

The description of the form of vibration just presented applies

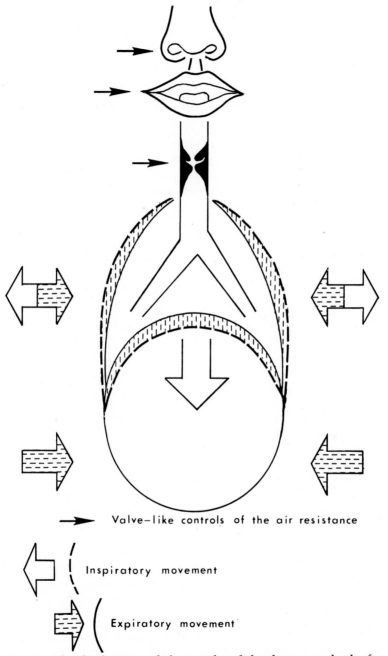

Valve—like controls of the air resistance

Inspiratory movement

Expiratory movement

Figure 3.   The diaphragm and the muscles of the thorax supply the force to distend the lungs and to displace the air. The airstream is controlled at several levels: the glottis, the articulatory organs, the nose. "From: De pathologische stembandfunctie Stafleu, Leiden Neth."

to the normal adult male voice (chest register). When frequency is raised the whole complex of the thyroarytenoid and lateral cricoarytenoid muscles is somewhat contracted, resulting in an increase of firmness of the vocal folds. The shortening that might result from this is compensated for by a moderate contraction of the cricothyroid muscles. The folds themselves are not only less supple, but also thinner, and the mass that is brought into vibration is less. Consequently this results in a lighter register which occurs in the higher male voice and which is also the normal mode of vibration for the adult female voice.

The production of a falsetto tone is entirely different. Cooker (1972) states:

> The falsetto register constitutes an entirely different mode of vibration for the glottal generator. The basic difference between the modal register and falsetto is the nature of the vibrating bodies. Whereas the entire shelf of muscular tissue vibrates in modal register, the rather thin vocal ligaments are the major vibrating elements in falsetto. This condition is produced by stretching the vocal ligaments, and at the same time, relaxing the muscles within the folds. Much greater tension (elasticity) is developed in the thin, passive ligaments than is possible in the more massive muscles of the body of the folds. Also, the effective mass of the vibrating body (vocal ligament) is quite small by comparison with the mass of the entire fold. Typically, the folds do not completely close during a vibratory cycle; consequently, the flow of air through the glottis is not interrupted abruptly and the resultant pressure disturbance is much smoother than it is in the modal register. The spectrum of the sound that is produced is characterized by a lack of energy in the higher harmonics and the resultant tone quality is readily perceived as different from that of the model register in the same individual (pp. 48-49).

The concept of *vocal registers* has long been of great interest to singing teachers as well as other disciplines concerned with normal and pathological sound production. Manuel Garcia and many others after him have spent a great deal of time and effort defining voice registers.

The normal male voice (chest register), the higher male voice (lighter register), and the falsetto voice (falsetto register) have already been mentioned in this chapter. All three registers are produced by laryngeal function and not from a type of "voice" resonating in the cavities of the chest and/or head. Nonetheless, there still appears to be confusion of terminology regarding the concept of registers.

The term chest register refers to the heavy, sonorous voice which sounds rattling in the lower ranges, metallic* in the high ranges, and which results from the abrupt explosions of air pressure that activate the resonance cavities above and below the glottis. The steep sound waves inside excite, in the resonance cavities, a large series of overtones from very high to very low. It is mainly the sudden closure of the glottis which imparts a sharp impulse to the air column in the oral and pharyngeal cavity.

Some confusion also exists with regard to the terms falsetto register and head register. Damsté (1968a) points out that with head voice we refer to the highest notes that can be produced with normal register. In his discussion of an article by Luchsinger (1949), it is stated that the vocal folds have been shown to be a few millimeters thicker when they are vibrating in normal register than when they are vibrating in falsetto and the vocal folds are shorter in head voice.

Regarding the glottis, or sound generator, the difference between the registers are as follows: chest register—soft, supple, thick vocal folds; falsetto register—thin, long, tense, stretched vocal ligaments with relaxed internal muscles (except the cricothyroid); head or midregister—shorter vocal folds, less stretching of the ligament, moderate firmness of the medial border of the vocal folds, and a larger mass of the folds participating in swinging than in falsetto.

The mid-register can be seen as a mixture of the chest and falsetto register. The mixing occurs by a simultaneous moderate contraction of the cricothyroid muscles (which stretch the vocal ligaments) and the vocalis muscles (which shorten the folds by

---

* Because there is no generally accepted nomenclature for the description of sound qualities, it is difficult to discuss this subject so that meanings are the same for all readers. It would be desirable to compare the perceived quality of the voice with acoustic properties of the sound wave with the form cf glottis vibration which produces the wave.

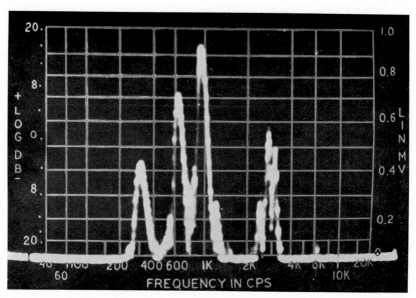

Figure 4A and B. Spectrograms of two voice sounds of the same fundamental frequency (290 Hz) in (A) normal register and (B) falsetto register. Remark the formant at 3000 Hz which is present in the normal clear voice and absent in the falsetto voice which is of a much poorer quality. "From: De pathologische stembandfunctie Stafleu, Leiden Neth."

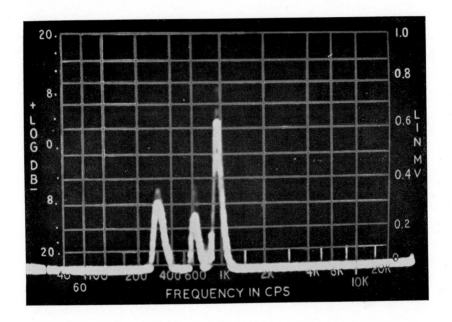

their contraction). The result is that the ligament is not fully stretched, and more lateral parts of the fold are coupled to the ligament and can participate in the vibration. The mass of the vocal fold is less flaccid, thus firmer, than in heavy or chest register. With controlled techniques of mixing registers there are no limits between separate registers. The article by Van den Berg (1968) contains an excellent discussion of the concept of register.

Timcke, von Leden, and Moore (1958, 1959) attempted to express the mode of glottis vibration in a ratio. This is the opening quotient: the duration of a lateral movement of the folds divided by the total duration of the vibration period; or the open quotient—the time during which the vocal folds are not in approximation to each other, divided by the total duration of the period. These quotients are, however, not easy to determine exactly because of the phase difference between the cranial and caudal parts of the vibrating folds. With the help of an electronic laryngostroboscope it is possible to get a global impression about the relation of the ratio of open and closed phase of the vibration. The open phase is short in chest register and long in falsetto register.

SUMMARY

The larynx, in its primary role of a sphincter, serves to protect the lower airway and to participate in the process of respiration. The function of phonation is secondary and, as is evidenced in the speech of the laryngectomized, can be accomplished without a larynx and with the simplest type of sphincter.

Many of the complexities of laryngeal functioning and its relation to sound production are still unknown. However, it is because of these complexities that there is a great variability of movement of the laryngeal structures which enable humans to produce a wide variety of voice sounds. It is through this ability that man is able to express his thoughts, feelings, and emotions (1) by the paralinguistic elements of speech (the speaking voice), and (2) by singing.

Like all complex devices the larynx is subject to breakdown. When sound production is disrupted the whole life of the person is affected. We are concerned with the factors that contribute to the dysfunction and with the restoration of the entire system.

Chapter 2

THE EXAMINATION AND DIAGNOSIS OF VOICE DISORDERS AND SPECIAL METHODS OF ACOUSTIC AND PHYSIOLOGIC RESEARCH

W HETHER IT IS A speech pathologist or a laryngologist who first sees the individual with a voice complaint, it will ultimately be both professionals who are responsible for a complete and thorough examination. The speech pathologist for the medical aspect of the examination will refer to the laryngologist, while most laryngologists, not being trained in speech pathology will, in turn, refer the patient to the speech pathologist for a more complete examination of the nonmedical areas of the complaint.

THE CASE HISTORY

As in every diagnostic examination, a complete and thorough case history is a necessity. A full discussion of procedures of history-taking is obviated here by the space limitation; however, there are a number of excellent references which will furnish the reader with procedures and techniques for interviewing. (Kinsey, Pomeroy, and Martin, 1948; Johnson, et al., 1963; Darley, 1964).

Many patients feel uneasy about supplying answers to questions that seem to have no connection with their primary complaint. If the interviewer can make the patient aware that answering all questions, no matter how tangential they may appear, will help make it easier to identify the problem so that a proper course of treatment can be recommended and a rapport may be established that will not only enhance the interview, but will be an asset to any therapeutic relationships that may continue. Darley (1964) states as follows:

> There is more to being an effective case-history taker than pleasantly asking questions. The interview constitutes a special kind of inter-action, a mutual viewing by two persons of one person's history. In the course of this interaction there develops a relationship-rapport which reduces the impedance to communicate. The informant becomes willing to divulge information when he sees in the inter-viewer a person whom he can respect and who can respect him, someone who understands his feelings and helps him cope with them, a person who knows what he is doing, who listens with care and discernment.

Regardless of whether the history is taken by the speech pathologist or the laryngologist, it should include such areas as the complaint as stated by the patient, pertinent identifying data, previous history of such a complaint, previous therapy (or therapies), the voice prior to the complaint, medical history, family history, family relationships, educational and vocational history, professional and social demands on the voice, etc. (Johnson, et al., 1963; Van Riper, 1963; and Berry and Eisenson, 1956 give examples of case history forms.)

The interviewer should be interested not only in gathering data for his form but should be observant of the patient's total behavior. How does he react to certain questions? Is there good eye contact with the interviewer? What type of facial expressions are seen, etc.? An interviewer whose "eyes and ears" are on his form alone will fail to collect all the pertinent data.

The interviewer must also concentrate on the patient's voice during the interview and make note of the observed particulars systematically: particulars about loudness, pitch, quality, etc.

The description of how the voice sounds is followed by observation about the way the voice is produced: signs of strain, excitement; depression; postural appearance; the way of breathing (high thoracic use of accessory respiratory musculature, normal or inverse movement of the abdominal wall). All aspects of vocal function are observed and recorded by the interviewer.

EXAMINATION OF THE FUNCTIONAL POSSIBILITIES
OF THE VOCAL MECHANISM

The central problem in the diagnosis of voice disorders is to determine the relative share of organic and functional factors in their genesis. Therefore, the patient is stimulated in different ways so as to provoke the most varied voice responses. (Moore, 1957, Chapter 22; and Darley, 1964, discuss various methods of voice testing and analysis.) Voice changes occurring on various instructions are observed: dry coughing, phonating when yawning, expiratory phonation afer a short inspiratory phonation, phonating during displacement and compression (lateral and in an a-p direction) of the larynx, phonating consecutively with a relaxed sigh, with a sharp metallic sound, in falsetto, etc. In this way the listener is able to concentrate on one aspect of voice at a time and is rapidly informed about (1) the functional possibilities of the organs, (2) the degree to which the patient has control over his vocal organs, and (3) his readiness and willingness to produce changes in his voice.

In all cases it is deemed of utmost importance to tape record the performance of each patient. This allows the examiner to recheck his initial impressions of the voice without undue attention to other factors, e.g. history-taking, maintaining conversation, etc. The recording can be utilized further with the patient to make him more aware of the abnormality and to provide the examiner an indication as to the patient's discriminative ability with regard to his disorder. Above all, the recording can serve as a lasting document to be kept for future comparison.

With some individuals the Lombard test could be administered. In this test a moderately loud noise (50 to 80 dB) is presented through earphones to both ears of the patient. When the noise is present, the patient will attempt to talk louder so as to hear himself. In the case of possible psychogenic voice disorder this may cause the voice quality to improve; in an organic disorder, the hoarseness will persist or deteriorate. Various other types of instrumentation have been used in attempting to analyze the aspects of pitch, quality, resonance, and loudness in an individual voice (Steer and Hanley, 1957,

Chapter 6). The utilization of some of this instrumentation will be discussed in a later section of this chapter.

LARYNGOLOGICAL EXAMINATION

The complexities of vocal disorders dictate that the examining physician be concerned not only about the laryngeal structure, but with the entire medical well-being of the individual. The voice disorder may merely serve as a sign to the physician that other, more serious, physical disorders exist.

The ear, nose, and throat (ENT) examination should include inspection of the oral and pharyngeal cavities for deviation and motility of the hard and soft palates, any existing dental abnormalities, movement and appearance of the tongue, etc. Although these areas may not be directly related to sound production, deviations may be indicative of other problems. An examination of the eardrums is also performed (in all instances the patient should have as complete an audiological work-up as may be needed in each case).

There should be an examination of the nose and the conductivity of both nasal passages separately. In addition, the physician will palpate the neck in a search for goitre; enlarged glands in the supraclavicular, cervical, and submaxillary region; and prominence and eventual displacement of the thyroid cartilage.

An indirect laryngoscopic examination should be performed. This laryngeal mirror examination is the visual inspection of the vocal folds, the ventricular folds, and the laryngeal entrance (epiglottic, arytenoids, and aryepiglottic folds). Low humming, dry cough, falsetto, piercing metallic sound on vowel, etc. will enable observation of the vocal folds during various functions, rather than in only one incidental position's belonging to a certain abnormal way of phonating. The examiner will thus be better able to conclude whether or not complete closure is possible, and that the separation or bowing of the folds may be due to a functional origin. (If the reader is further interested in the total examination for voice disorders Luchsinger and Arnold, 1965, have presented an outline for a phoniatric examination.)

DIAGNOSIS AND TREATMENT

Once the examiner has appraised the problem in terms of all his findings and all the alternative possibilities, he must then make a differential diagnosis. However, if his findings indicate the need for further referral (psychiatric, psychological, neurological, etc.) then the diagnosis must be delayed until the entire appraisal of the patient has been completed.

In any case, in voice pathology it is usually not possible to express the diagnosis in a single word or simple statement. Rather, many dimensions have to be accounted for: (1) the organic state of the larynx with its possibilities and its limitations; (2) the constitutional situation of the organism, its strength and weakness; (3) the psychogenic or habitual factor that has led to the disturbed function and that is maintaining it; and (4) the factors existing in the environment.

Thus a complete diagnosis in a certain case might be put on record as: habitual hyperkinetic dysphonia with proliferative laryngitis in a middle-aged salesman, athletic type, heavy smoker, moderate drinker, with anxiety about his job. Were the same case to be put on record as: proliferative laryngitis of posterior part of the left cord, this would give an insufficient picture of the person, the situation, the prognosis, and the indicated treatment.

Finally, a therapy program is prescribed, based on all the available information. Therapy can consist of:

1. Improvement of the organic conditions by surgical intervention (removing a polyp, draining and rinsing an empyeme of a maxillary sinus).
2. Pharmaceutical treatment of constitutional defects, deficiencies, or bodily dysequilibrium (sedative, hormonal agent).
3. Modifying a noxious function (exercises for relaxation, breath control, voice therapy).
4. Improving circumstantial or situational conditions (talking with employer or relatives) or desensitizing the patient to the provocative factors in his environment.

In most cases the above-cited program of interviewing and examination will suffice for appraisal of the voice complaint. For certain cases, however, the examination will have to be supplemented with other methods of objective measurement.

SPECIAL METHODS OF ACOUSTIC AND PHYSIOLOGIC RESEARCH

Because many assumptions derived from clinical practice have yet to be scientifically tested, subjective notation by the examiner of the loudness, pitch, and quality of the voice should be supplemented by objective measurements. This is not always possible in the clinical situation and must, therefore, for the present be confined to the research laboratory. This stresses the need for greater cooperation between the laryngologist and the voice pathologist. In the final analysis, diagnosis and treatment will be based not merely upon the results obtained in the research laboratory, but also upon what the *individual* examiner *sees* and *hears* in his examination of the patient.

Briefly, some methods of objective assessment are:

1. Recording the sound intensity, the fundamental frequency, and the quality of the sound.
2. Stroboscopic laryngoscopy.
3. Estimating or measuring vocal fold length.
4. X-ray examination of the vocal mechanism.
5. Electromyography.
6. Measuring the respiratory capacity, the breathing movements and the respiratory airflow.

Recording the Sound Intensity, the Fundamental Frequency and the Quality of the Sound

Sound Intensity

It is known that there can be a difference as great as 70 dB between the "softest" sound an individual can produce and the loudest vocalization he can produce. One of the simplest ways of measuring sound intensity is with a microphone, amplifier, and AC voltmeter combination. With the addition of a calibrated attenuator and frequency-weighting network, this simple instrument now becomes a decibelmeter or sound-level meter. The sound pressure can be read directly in the dB above an internationally determined zero level. The reader will find the discussion by Steer and Hanley (1957, Chapter 6) much more detailed.

The sensitivity for various frequencies (transmission curve) can be adjusted. If such an instrument and method are to be used, it is important that the conditions of testing always be the same, meaning the room in which the testing is done, the distance to the microphone, and other factors which may influence the results. A simple system that is used clinically is one in which the intensity and the frequency of the sound can be plotted against each other in a graph, resulting in a clear diagram of the frequency range and range of intensity, which we have called the "fonetogram" (Waar and Damsté, 1968).

Fundamental Frequency

It would be difficult, indeed, in a clinical situation to utilize the varied instrumentation available for the measurement of fundamental frequency (repetition rate of the vocal folds). Of course, one could attempt to use a simple pitch or frequency indicator, but like the human ear, this instrument may make errors. In some sharp metallic sounds, for instance, a dominating harmonic may be chosen instead of a weak fundamental. The terms frequency and pitch have become so interlinked with one another that there is a tendency for people to use them synonymously. As pointed out by Fry (1968), "As far as the pitch of speech sounds is concerned, we may take it that in direct communcation through the air the fundamental of voiced sounds is generally audible and is the chief correlate of pitch."

Because of the correlation between pitch and frequency, determining the pitch of the voice should not be difficult for anybody with a musical ear if he is able to compare the produced tone with a calibrated source of sound. This source of sound must be able to produce a series of tones from 60 to 1600 Hz. A sine tone generator is not suitable because the sound is not com-

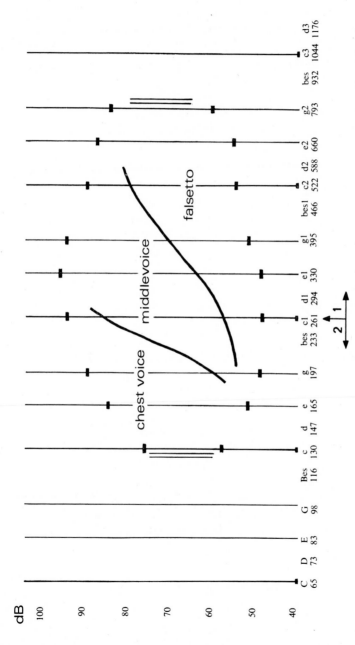

Figure 5. Phonetogram. By plotting the minimal and maximal intensity of each tone that can be produced, a field is traced which marks out the voice range and the intensity span.

parable with the complex sound of the human voice. A har-
monium, chordetta, or electronic organ is very suitable, provided
the tuning is reliably calibrated. Further examples and descrip-
tions of instrumentation used in determining fundamental frequency can be found in Fry (1968, Chapter 12), and Michel,
et al. (1966).

Quality of the Sound

Quality has been defined from an acoustical point of view,
as "Quality: when applied to voice, the acoustic characteristics
of vowels resulting from their overtone structure or the relative
intensities of their frequency components" (Wood, 1957).

From a perceptual point of view, quality is a highly subjective
concept. Essentially two methods can be applied to determining
quality acoustically: (1) harmonic analysis and (2) describing
the characteristics of an impulse-period in time.

In order to perform a harmonic analysis, one would utilize an
instrument intended for calculating the number of partials in any
given tone along with the relative intensities. The general
principle of harmonic analysis is to allow sound to pass through a
series of filters and to make a record of the level of the signal
that is passed by each filter. The visual image depends, among
other things, on the number and the band-width of the filters used.

Harshness or hoarseness is determined partly by nonperiodic
phenomena such as irregular intervals between impulses and
super-position of noise on top of the impulses. These phenomena
are not accessible utilizing the above-mentioned analysis. Studies
in the analysis of hoarseness have been carried out by Michel
(1964), Moore and Thompson (1965), and Coleman and Wendahl
(1967). An acoustic and methodical analysis of the direct oscillo-
gram can provide a more precise acoustic description. Attempts
have been made to correlate this with the perceptual description
of the sound.

Stroboscopy of the Larynx

Stroboscopic examination of the vocal folds is the use of
indirect laryngoscopy together with an intermittent flashing of
light. This type of approach enables the examiner to see the

vibrating folds as if in a stationary position or moving at a very slow rate.

This is due in part to the fact that the vibrations are periodical. The vibrating folds are illuminated with an intermittent source of light. When the frequencies of the vibrating folds and the light flashes are equal, a continuous image of the folds standing still in one phase of vibration is seen; by changing the phase of the intermittent source of light, all phases of vibration can be studied. However, the light flashes have to run precisely synchronously with the vocal fold vibration. When their frequency is lowered slightly and they are not tuned exactly, there will be a continuous change of phase. The light flash will hit each vibration period at a somewhat later phase and the vibrations of the folds will appear to be occurring at a very slow rate.

The principle of stroboscopy (discovered by Plateau in 1833) was first applied for the observation of vocal fold vibration in the second half of the nineteenth century. In the older instrumentation, the flashing light source was achieved by means of a disc containing holes which rotated in front of an existing light source. The number of flashes per second was controlled by the rate of revolution of the disc. Synchronization of the light flashes and the vocal folds vibration is possible only with a subject capable of maintaining a tone on an exact pitch. Even then the continuously changing phase relation between the vibrations and the flashes may produce a source of error in the observation. Van den Berg (1968) has an excellent discussion of the possible sources of error in stroboscopic examination.

A great improvement in stroboscopic instrumentation was the generation of light flashes by a gas discharge tube controlled by a microphone. This helped to facilitate the examination and to make it more reliable. While the patient phonates at different pitches, the frequency of the light flashes is controlled by the vocal fold vibration via the microphone. However, in achieving one advantageous aspect, a disadvantage is introduced: this continuous synchronization does not allow the observer to view the vocal folds in a very slow rate of vibration. Additions to the instrumentation allow the examiner to turn a knob manually through all the phases of one period and return. This, however, does not give a picture of continuous motion, and the speed of vibration is dependent upon the speed of turning.

Van den Berg (1958) has designed a circuitry, the delta-f generator, which lowers the frequency of the light flashes in relation to the frequency of the vocal folds. The difference is adjustable between 0.2 and 2 Hz. This device has made the stroboscope a much more suitable instrument for clinical practice by allowing the examiner to view a whole range of voice productions without having to make laborious and time-consuming adjustments. Further details about stroboscopy and the instrumentation involved have been thoroughly discussed by Winckel (1965).

Reliable use of the stroboscope in clinical practice has existed only for a short time. Several symptoms have been described in the older literature which are no longer evident with modern equipment. We can only conclude that these were the consequences of observation with inferior equipment.

The stroboscopic examination of the vocal folds is done in the same way as was the ordinary indirect laryngoscopy: with a perforated headmirror and a larynx mirror. The normal lamp is replaced by the xenon-flashtube of the stroboscope. The vocal folds present their uppersurface, the medial surfaces that are directed towards each other are partly visible during the open phase of the vibration. This is definitely an advantage over ordinary laryngoscopy. In ordinary laryngoscopy the rapid vibration during phonation blurs the medial borders, and small irregularities may be hidden from the examiner's view. However, in stroboscopic light the vibration parts of the larynx are seen clearly and sharply and any protusions of the medial surfaces of the vocal folds are clearly defined.

The Normal Vibration Pattern

The circulating wave of vibration energy is observed from above as a movement to and fro. The parting of the vocal folds is called the opening phase and the coming together the closing phase. The ratio of the open phase to the total duration of the period is the open quotient. This can be large, as in head voice and falsetto, or small, as in the chest register (long closed phase).

The smaller the open quotient, the more harmonic are the overtones generated with the fundamental.

The maximal swinging movement of vibrating folds is called amplitude. This is larger in chest register than in falsetto. Because the very fast vibration in well-adjusted stroboscopic light appears as a quietly undulating movement, every detail of the vibration can be observed. The consistency of the fold which is controlled by the tonus of the intrinsic laryngeal muscles and the stretching of the ligaments can be appraised.

Estimating or Measuring Vocal Fold Length

Because the range and the type of voice are known to be correlated with the length of the vocal folds, it is important in some instances to express this in a quantifiable manner. The experienced laryngologist can, with the naked eye, discern between folds of great, medium, and small length. However, more objective methods are to (1) use a laryngeal mirror upon which is etched the form of a pattern of one milimeter squares, or (2) use the method suggested by Zimmerman (1938) in which the mirror image is reflected by means of a semipermanent mirror and is observed by a second examiner against a black background containing a calibrated scale. Although this is liable to cause error and is somewhat cumbersome another method (3) of measuring vocal fold length (although exact measurements should not be expected from this method) is use of cinematographic or X-ray techniques. Practical procedures have been indicated by Hollien and others (1968, 1962, 1960a, 1960b).

In the earlier studies (1960) in which high-speed cinematography was used, it was revealed that in the abducted position the length of the glottis ranged from 19.1 to 23 mm. There was a notable decrease in the length, ranging from 18 mm to 20.5 mm, when the subject phonated various pitches going from low to high tones, but not including falsetto. They also noted that as pitch became higher the length of the vocal folds increased. In other studies utilizing X-ray techniques (Hollien and Curtis, 1960; Hollien, 1962, 1964; Hollien, Coleman, and Moore, 1968) it was noted that as the fundamental frequency increased there was an associated decrease in the thickness of the vocal folds and an increase in their length.

It is highly recommended that the reader investigate these references to obtain more precise information on the relationship of vocal fold length to fundamental frequency.

X-ray Examination of the Larynx

The examination by laryngeal mirror allows the examiner to view the larynx only from above. Since other dimensions are of equal importance for diagnostic purposes, the laryngeal examination can be supplemented by the a-p and the lateral X-ray exposures of the neck. Damsté (1968) supplies a thorough discussion of the clinical application of the many X-ray studies.

In the a-p exposure, the difficulty encountered is that the vocal folds do not stand out clearly against the heavy shadow of the cervical vertebral column. There are several solutions for this problem:

1. Tomography—Frontal tomograms of a cross section or preset slice of the larynx yield a far sharper exposure of the larynx (true and false vocal folds, etc.) by making the other structures more indistinct through exposure time and other factors.

2. Laryngography—This is another radiological investigation in which, after surface anasthesia of the mucosa, a fluid contrast medium is sprayed over the epithelium. In this way the contours of the vestibules of the larynx, as well as other anatomical details of the larynx, appear clearly marked on the film. Laryngography is of great importance, especially for the evaluation of the subglottic region, in the case of tumor growth. For a more thorough and complete discussion of laryngography and its comparison to other procedures, the reader is referred to Landman (1966a).

3. Translation—This is a method in which the larynx is pushed sidewards so that its shadow is projected next to the shadow of the vertebral column. On the translation X-ray, as well as the tomogram, the muscle complex of the vocal folds and the ventricular folds appears between the ven-

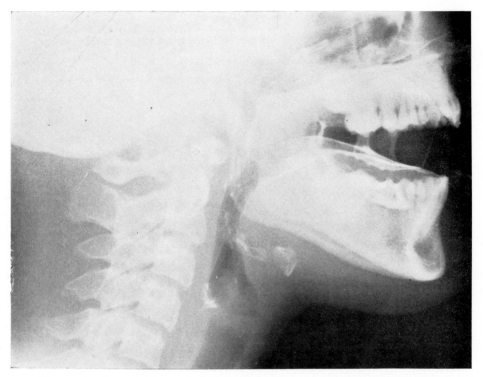

Figure 6. Lateral Xray of the neck and low facial part of the skull. Compare with Figure 1. Note the base of the skull and vertebral column from C₁ to C₇; the lumen of the trachea, the larynx, the pharynx, and the oral and nasal cavities; the vocal fold, the arytenoid, the epiglottis, the hyoid bone; the base, dorsum, and apex of the tongue; the soft palate; the lower and upper jaw with the teeth.

tricle of Morgagni. Form and thickness of the folds in various sorts of phonation can be clearly discerned.

By means of a lateral Xray a survey of the voice generator and the entire vocal tract is obtained. The most pronounced parts and contours of the vocal tract that can be recognized are the base of the skull, the cervical vertebral column from C1 to C7; the lumen of the trachea, larynx, pharynx, and oral cavity; the vocal folds, arytenoids, epiglottis, and hyoid bone; the base, dorsum, and the apex of the tongue; the soft palate; and the mandible and maxilla with their elements.

The following features are of special importance for voice function: the curvature (lordosis, kyphosis) of the vertebral column; the level of the larynx as related to the axis of the cervical vertebral column (this determines the length of the vocal tract); the length of the vocal folds; the width of the pharynx and oral cavity.

Electromyography

Recording the action potentials in groups of contracting muscle fibers has its most important application in cases of afflictions of the peripheral neuron. This method is also applied in physiological voice research to record contraction of normal muscles with voice and speech production. Excellent reviews of electromyographic investigations of laryngeal muscles are referred to the reader in Faaborg-Andersen (1957); Brewer, Briess, and Faaborg-Andersen (1960); Buchthal and Faaborg-Andersen (1960); and Faaborg-Andersen and Vennard (1964).

Measuring the Respiratory Capacity, the Breathing Movements, and the Respiratory Airflow

Pneumonography

Pneumography is a way of analyzing respiratory movements. The instrumentation available for such analysis can be either of the pneumatic or electronic type. In either device the rate and extent of the individual's breathing movements (inhalation-exhalation of the thorax and the abdomen) are recorded graphically.

Spirography

In general there are two types of spirometers, wet and dry, but the dry type is not as reliable as the wet. In both types the air volume which is displaced by the respiratory organ is measured. A simple wet spirometer consists of a cylinder closed on top, floating in water, and contained in a larger cylinder. The subject blows through a tube into the cylinder, which is forced upward by the air. The height to which the inner cylinder is lifted is a measure of the displaced volume of air. If a system of counterweights, a writing pen, graph paper, and a revolving drum are attached to this apparatus the displaced volume can be recorded on a graph. Spirograms are used for evaluation of lung function such as vital capacity, which is the greatest amount of air an individual can exhale after his maximum amount of inhalation; complementary air, which is that amount of air that can still be drawn in after a normal inspiration; and reserve air, which is that amount of air that can be expired after a normal expiration. (A detailed account of pneumography and spirography, techniques and research, can be found in Steer and Hanley, 1957).

Pneumotachography

This method is used to measure and record the speed of the airflow during phonic respiration. The most frequently used instrumentation is the pneumotachograph designed by Fleisch (1933). It has been applied mostly in physiological research in voice function and for physical description of deviant forms of voice production. For clinical purposes there are ways to determine the approximate usage of air during phonation that give a practical indication of the efficiency of the voice production. The *maximal phonation time* amounts, for males, to a mean of thirty-five seconds, for females twenty-six seconds, with large individual differences. The extreme values (outside the 95 percentile) are longer than sixty-two seconds in the male, forty in the female, and shorter than fifteen seconds (male) or fourteen seconds (female). The latter values may be considered clinically abnormal. These data are taken from Hirano Koike and Von Leden (1968) as well as the following:

$$\text{phonation quotient} = \frac{\text{vital capacity}}{\text{maximal phonation time}}$$

More than 307 ml/sec for the male, or 241 ml/sec for the female may be considered abnormal. The phonation quotient is much easier to determine than the mean flow rate and shows a high correlation with it, as tested by the above-mentioned authors.

Measuring Pressure in the Thoracic and Abdominal Cavities

Measurement of pressure in the thoracic and abdominal cavities can be accomplished by utilization of pressure receptors which are introduced into the esophagus or the stomach via the nose or mouth. In certain conditions the pressure in the esophagus is equal to the subglottic pressure in the trachea. The pressure in the stomach is used as a measure for the pressure under the diaphragm. In this way an attempt is made to determine what part the diaphragm has in controlling the subglottic pressure.

By the utilization of the previously mentioned methods it is possible to give a much more objective description of the many variables which are important in voice production. All the research employing these methods have added greatly to our knowledge of normal and pathological voice production and can contribute to a more correct diagnosis and treatment.

Chapter 3

DISORDERS OF MUTATION

ONE OF THE MOST striking features of the human voice is the large difference between the male and female voices. The pitch and the quality of the voice is a sexual characteristic and of great importance in personal relations, although we usually do not focus attention upon it unless there is a deviation from the normal, such as a man with a high-pitched voice or a woman with a baritone voice.

It is the examiner's task to determine the degree of the organic and/or functional nature of the disturbance. The mean pitch of a man is lower than that of a woman. We can see, however, that there is a great area of overlap for the male and female voice. In most cases, even within that area, one is able to recognize the sex of the speaker because this is not only characterized by pitch, but also by the sound quality. However, the sound quality can also vary within wide limits.

From an organic point of view, every healthy voice organ has a large range of vocal possibilities. When organic pathology is present, these limits will be noticeably restricted. Most mutational disturbances in young men are not of organic origin. However, an organic pathology is present in cases of virilization of the female voice.

SEXUAL MATURATION

One phase of growth is known as puberty. This phase occurs between the age of twelve to fifteen years. The bodily meta-

39

morphoses and the changes of physiological function are considerable. There is a strong period of growth and the development of sexual maturation. In the young male this means that the hormones of the anterior lobe of the hypophysis cause the production of testosterone in the sexual glands to increase strongly within a short time period. Under the influence of this androgenic substance, the sexual organs develop into fully functioning organs (testes, prostatic glands, and vesicles). Also, other bodily characteristics (secondary sex characteristics) develop under the influence of androgenic hormones during puberty: hair growth in different places, change in proportions and in the voice due to a considerable and unproportional growth of the larynx by which the vocal folds can increase to one and a half times their length. This is especially true in boys. In girls the transition to sexual maturity (the beginning of the ovulation and the menstruation cycles) is expressed mainly in alterations of body contour, with change of the voice, although present, less striking.

The changes in puberty can be retarded or absent altogether if the hypophysis does not produce its hormones at the right moment (hypophyseal hypogonadism) or by castration or atrophy of the sexual glands (eunochoidism). The delay of voice change by one of these endocrine developmental disturbances is, however, a rare occurrence.

NORMAL COURSE OF VOICE CHANGE IN MALES

Mutation of the voice normally occurs between twelve and fifteen years of age and is characterized by a period of hoarseness which lasts several months. On close observation the hoarseness appears to consist of rapid fluctuations of the voice quality between the chest and the falsetto registers. This has sometimes been referred to as voice or pitch breaks. The instability of the voice is typical of males in puberty. As long as this continues laryngeal examination reveals a diffuse redness of the vocal folds and an incomplete closure of the posterior commissure. Curry, in his article "Hoarseness and Voice Change in Male Adolescents" (1949) discusses this aspect.

The following data are derived from a systematical investigation of 100 Czechoslovakian boys between the ages of eleven and fifteen years (Naidr, et al. 1965): (1) The mutation process has a mean duration of thirteen months. (2) The greatest changes of the voice occur in the thirteenth, fourteenth, and fifteenth year. (3) The voice changes begin a short time before the growth of the larynx and manifest themselves first in the singing voice— the upper limit of the range is lowered and the lower tones become unstable. The vocal range is somewhat reduced. Later, the lowering of the voice is followed by an increase of the range. The speaking voice is lowered during the mutation with a mean of eight semitones. The mutation, however, is not only a change in the vocal range, but above all a change in voice quality. The heavy register of the adult male voice takes the place of the lighter register of the boy's voice.

VOICE DISORDERS IN RELATION TO THE MUTATION

The Mutation Falsetto

The mutation falsetto is not the result of an organic disorder. Rather it is the habitual use of falsetto voice in males whose laryngeal growth has been normal and who exhibit the ability to produce the normal chest voice of the adult male. Although its prevalence in the population is not great, the high-pitched female voice in the adult male is a striking phenomenon which usually calls attention to itself. However, not everybody is acquainted with the fact that the disturbances in many cases can be corrected rather simply. The most suitable time would be in the early stages of this disorder. The patients who have been seen for this vary in age from fifteen to fifty-eight years of age, with 50 percent being over twenty years of age. With such a disorder one can only hypothesize the etiological factors involved.

1. These boys are said to be shy, bashful, passive, or exhibit feminine behavior. This might influence their choice in a direction of a nonvirile, more childish type of voice. In

reverse, however, the possession of such a voice might cause such behavior.

2. The environment, in this case the relation to the parents and the place in the family, frequently appears to be a point of importance. In other words, has the individual been able at that point in the maturational process to accept the role of an adult male?

3. In more than a few cases the chest register of the patient sounded rather heavy and the period of mutation occurred at a relatively young age compared to his peers. It could be assumed that such a boy may have continued to use his falsetto voice so that he would not be considered "different" from the other boys in his age group. After a short while the habitual use of such a voice can become fixed and the normal adult chest register is not used.

Parallel incidence of some of these factors may be sufficient to lead to a deviation. Continued use of such voice quality is its prime maintaining factor. There is an obstinate misunderstanding that the mutation falsetto is a disturbance of endocrine origin, a consequence of sexual immaturity. Even in professional literature traces of this unjust opinion are still found. It is misleading to treat the voice disturbance in relation to mutation under the area of endocrine voice disturbances, as sometimes happens. Mutation is, of course, a hormonally determined event, but the voice disturbance is not. This is true for the prolonged mutation, the mutation falsetto, and the incomplete mutation. In these cases it is usually not due to hormonal regulation that the patient has emerged from puberty with an abnormal voice. Here the sexual development has been followed by an abnormal functional adaptation, as far as the use of the voice is concerned.

It is obvious to any observer that these boys are not exceptional in any way as to their secondary sex characteristics. Facial growth and skin eruptions, like acne, are already indications of androgenic hormonal activity. The laryngeal prominence (Adam's Apple) and the laryngoscopic image also point to a completely full-grown larynx. It is not generally recognized that the high voice in itself may serve as proof that sexual development has taken place; the falsetto voice appears to be different from the young boy's voice and is characterized by its weak quality and small dynamic range. In a study by Duffy and Lerman (1970) it was noted that listeners could consistently recognize the high-pitched voice of children when compared to the falsetto voices of adult males.

The case history often reveals vocal deviation during puberty. It is usually stated that there are voice "breaks," but that later the voice tends to remain at a high-pitched level. Some patients are also well aware that they are capable of producing a low voice. They have rejected this because it seems rather "heavy and strange."

On examination a normal full-grown larynx is found with a visible and palpable Adam's Apple. Laryngoscopic examination confirms this, revealing fully developed vocal folds. The most important aspect of the examination is the proper evaluation of the voice function. Sometimes a cough, laugh, or other involuntary vocal act shows that a low sound is within the vocal possibilities. If not, the examiner must attempt to induce a low sound with various instructions and manipulations.

Now and then some organic abnormalities have been noted in some individuals with this type of vocal quality: (1) a paralyzed vocal fold; (2) history of struma operation; (3) slight retardation of skeletal age (according to radiologic findings). In all three instances where such organic abnormality was noted, treatment resulted in a completely normal voice quality.

Treatment of Mutation Falsetto Voice

With a normal vocal organ it is possible to produce a normal male voice. In the habitual falsetto voice, the larynx is often in a cranial position with the cricoid and thyroid approximated by the contracted cricothyroid muscles. Exactly the reverse position is taken in yawning. The clinician, therefore, should make use of such an action in treatment. In an erected posture of the trunk and a wide thorax, the diaphragm is flattened and the base of the tongue is displaced in a caudal direction. This posture increases the pulling force to the trachea which promotes shortening of the vocal folds. This shortening is enhanced with manipulation of the larynx by placing the thumb on the notch of the thyroid cartilage and pushing the larynx in a dorsal and caudal direction. It is preferred that the patient "pull" his own larynx down with his own musculature and that the thumb only acts as a reminder.

If a more normal pitch is achieved with just the yawning action, the clinician should continue to use this method until the patient is very consistent and appears to be unembarrassed by and used to the new voice. When the new voice is fairly well-established using this method, the patient can then proceed, very mechanically, through nonsense syllables, counting words, etc. In each consecutive step there is always a possibility that old vocal habits will reoccur. If this happens, the clinician should return to that point in therapy where the patient can consistently produce the more normal vocal pitch.

The reaction of patients to the new sound is very different. Some are very enthusiastic and completely accepting, others are embarrassed and do not like the new sound, while still others are literally shocked and resist any change. Based on the patient's reaction and resistance or compliance with therapy, treatments can be as few as one with full success, too many with little or no success. A most remarkable history is that of a fifty-eight-year-old patient with a falsetto voice:

> The patient was fifty-eight years of age and was treated since his sixteenth birthday by various physicians for the problem of falsetto voice. After many, many years of unsuccessful medical treatment the patient consulted a "quack." His advice was for the patient to gargle his own urine. This therapy program, after some hesitation, was followed faithfully. This was also not successful. Many years later, when the patient was fifty years of age, he received three months of voice therapy with a speech clinician. Although his articulation habits improved, his voice did not change. Years later the man consulted one of the authors (Damsté). Examination revealed a normal laryngeal structure. In laughing and in phonating during laryngoscopy a more normal sound could be heard. With manipulation of the larynx and mechanical vibration applied to the sternum the patient was able to consistently produce a low voice, within a ten-minute period. Another ten minutes of exercise without manipulation and vibration showed that the patient could sustain

the new voice. After this single treatment the patient's voice has never gone back into falsetto, except once in an emotionally laden telephone conversation. The man, in a later follow-up, reported that upon his arrival home, after his initial visit, he continued to use his new voice. His grandchildren were very much amazed and then later uttered their disappointment that grandfather now had a voice like everybody else; previously he was considered as a special person because of his "fine" voice. His wife was also disappointed, however, for another reason. Why hadn't he consulted her? His answer, that he didn't expect any satisfactory results, did not satisfy her. Two days later she stated, "I wish you had your old voice back."

The Prolonged Mutation

The instability of the voice and the alternating of high and low pitch is considered characteristic for the voice in puberty, although it does not necessarily occur in all boys. The change in voice can occur so gradually that voice breaks may occur so seldom that it goes unnoticed. In individuals with prolonged mutation, pitch breaks occur to such a degree and over such a prolonged period that it is considered a nuisance and abnormal. If, after six months to a year, the instability of the voice does not decrease, it can safely be said that the limits of normal have been exceeded. In prolonged mutation, as contrasted to mutation falsetto, the voice is not constantly high, but alternates between high and low pitch. In some cases the high voice may dominate, with the voice breaking downwards in the accentuated syllables.

Not much value can be attached to the terminology that the patient uses to describe his own voice. He often refers to his low voice, which impresses us as normal, as hoarse. It would appear as if he has some negative feeling for the lower sound. When he says "sometimes I have a hoarse voice," it could possibly be interpreted as "sometimes I have a strange low voice which I find disagreeable."

A twenty-year-old male, married and in the military service, reported that his low voice "sounded so vulgar." In therapy he was able to produce the more normal adult pitch at will, but in spontaneous speech his high voice tended to dominate. He related that when he first began to use his low voice at home, his wife reacted strangely. She then was invited to attend the next therapy session. Through discussion with the therapist the wife was better able to understand the problem and agreed that the low voice was much more desirable. The husband also reported that he was a very timid person, that he often allowed his wife to do the talking for him while he preferred to speak softly and with his high voice. Through continued therapy, counseling and new insights, and changed role of the wife, he now uses a normal male adult pitch in spontaneous speech and appears to have taken on a more masculine role.

The Incomplete Mutation

In this disorder the individual has failed to develop normal adult male pitch and voice quality, although the physical mutation seems to have been completed and sexual development is normal. The voice lacks normal chest resonance, is somewhat dull and high-pitched, but not falsetto. The register break, typical of mutation falsetto, is not found in this disorder. Usually the period of mutation has passed relatively unnoticed. This is expressed in the German term, "larvierte mutation" (Zumsteeg, 1916), which means that during the changes of the voice organ in puberty, voice function did not attain full development.

What etiological factors are responsible for this lack of vocal development? The answer, as yet, is not fully known. An analysis of many cases has indicated a wide variety of etiological possibilities. On laryngoscopy the vocal folds appear slightly parted in the middle (oval glottis). This can be explained by an incompetence of the adductors (the lateral cricothyroid muscles). Failure of this muscle causes the arytenoid not to tilt downwards sufficiently so as to relax the conus elasticus completely. Thus a normal chest register is not possible (Chapter 1). The case histories suggest that tense and uncontrolled breathing habits contribute to the development of incomplete mutation. This voice appears to be more prevalent in people who have suffered from bronchitis, asthma, and other problems of the respiratory tract. The prognosis is not optimistic because the poor respiratory habits and lack of voice control have been well-established and in turn have led to some organic structural changes which cannot be overcome without drastic reeducation measures, if at all. Therapy consists of training breath control and the right degree of glottal closure during phonation.

Chapter 4

FUNCTIONAL DYSPHONIA

T HE QUALITY OF the voice depends upon a delicate balance between glottic closure and breath flow. Emotions can easily have a disturbing influence upon this balance. "Voice has often been called the barometer of the emotions" (Van Riper and Irwin, 1958). Various emotions in the individual may arouse changes in his physiological as well as psychological state. Eisenson, et al., (1963) state:

> When the emotional reactions are more intense, we are likely to become aware of the specifics of the physiological changes. We may then become aware of physical (muscular) tenseness, of heart palpitations, dryness of the throat, panting, heavy breathing, sweating and even changes in body temperature (p. 70).

Of prime importance to sound production are changes in physical tenseness and respiratory patterns. Significant changes in muscular tension (of hypo- or hyperfunction) may cause a disturbance of the delicate balance between subglottic pressure, breath flow, and glottal resistance (firmness of closure).

THE HYPO- AND HYPERKINETIC SYNDROMES

It seems obvious from previous discussion that voice disorders can occur without the vocal apparatus' being affected organically in any way. Although terminology in voice disorders may differ slightly, functional pathology can be considered to exist primarily in two syndromes with various subcategories. These are the hypokinetic syndrome and the hyperkinetic syndrome. The major vocal symptoms of the hypokinetic syndrome is breathiness due to insufficient closure of the vocal folds, lack of chest resonance, and poor projection of the voice. For the hyperkinetic syndrome the pathology consists of a too firmly constricted glottis, resulting in harshness and hoarseness.

FUNCTIONAL DYSPHONIA

Included in this category are those voice disturbances in which the organic condition of the vocal apparatus is not a primary factor. In other words, these are voice disorders which exist without any known organic pathology.

Breathiness

Fairbanks (1960) has stated that "breathy quality is almost invariably accompanied by limited vocal intensity . . . vocal attacks tend to aspirate . . ." Due to lack of proper glottal closure there is an escape of excessive air through the glottis. The familiar breathy voice of certain females has a functional origin, although in some instances breathiness is organic in nature. As previously stated, breathiness is the major symptom of the hypokinetic syndrome.

Breathy voice quality is, in all likelihood, a learned voice quality. Breathiness, as a nonorganic vocal quality, does not receive great attention from the laryngologist or the speech pathologist since it is generally accepted by the public as a symbolization of femininity.

Harshness

Harshness has been defined as a rough, raspy voice that is generally unpleasant to the ear. Other characteristics associated with the individual with a hoarse voice quality are rapid articulation, monotony, low pitch, reduced pitch range, and in some instances glottal or vocal fry. Fairbanks (1960) has referred to harshness as ". . . irregular aperiodic noise in the vocal fold spectrum . . . such speakers often overuse the extremely low pitches in their vocal areas, where maximum intensity is relatively low. Harsh speakers tend to initiate phonations abruptly with obtrusive glottal attacks."

Although Rees (1958) found no statistically significant evidence "of a relationship between abruptness of vowel initiation and degree of perceived harshness," she did present enough conclusive evidence to support the thesis that the obtrusive glottal attack is associated with harshness. In an earlier study (1958a) Rees indicated that perceived harshness changes in relation to a number of variables.

Many people feel that vocal fry is part of the total problem of harshness. Previously it has been considered as a vocal disorder in and of itself. Recently, however, research (Hollien, 1966) has indicated that "vocal fry involves a physiologically normal mode of laryngeal operation that results in a distinctive acoustic signal." Hollien and Michel (1968) reported that the fundamental frequency of vocal fry is far below that of the modal phonatory register. Male subjects in that study had a frequency range from 7 to 78 Hz for vocal fry, and for female subjects the range was from 2 to 78 Hz. The research concerned with this phenomenon (Coleman, 1963; Wendahl, Moore and Hollien, 1963; Michel and Hollien, 1968; and Hollien and Michel, 1968) points to the fact that it is a separate phonational register which results from periodic repetition rates of the folds. Therefore, it can exist as a separate entity, but can also be present as a vocal pathology, such as in harshness.

Another concept of harshness related to the definition by Fairbanks (1960) is that of aperiodicity. Zemlin feels (1968) that "the feature which differentiates the normal from the harsh voice is aperiodic noise, or irregular vocal fold vibration, which is often due to excessive tension of the folds." Wendahl (1966) has used the terms "jitter" and "shimmer" in his investigation of the concept of aperiodicity or roughness of the voice. Jitter is referred to as the "abrupt cycle-to-cycle frequency variation" or "the rapid random variations in fundamental frequency." "When the amplitude level of adjacent pulses were alternately attenuated, the resulting amplitude varying signal was termed shimmer." Based on the definition by Fairbanks and the results of the studies (Wendahl, 1966; Coleman and Wendahl, 1967), the judgment of harshness and/or hoarseness will be more likely as the aperiodic component of the vocal output increases.

Harshness does not occur only as a functional disorder of the voice. "The most revealing difference between functional harshness and harshness caused by organic change is the greater persistence of the latter. The function problem tends to disappear during shouting, laughing, increased breath flow, and general relaxed situation; the quality when caused by pathologic conditions is less variable" (Moore, 1971). The etiology of functional harshness is considered to be due to excessive force caused by tension in the various laryngeal muscle groups.

Hoarseness

Various terms, such as strained, coarse, raspy, etc., have been used in describing hoarseness. Fairbanks (1960) describes hoarseness as combining "the features of harshness and breathiness." In most instances this disorder is usually associated with severe colds or laryngitis. However, it may also be a symptom of diseases such as carcinoma, tuberculosis, and syphilis; therefore, it is of extreme importance that an individual presenting such a symptom be subjected to laryngoscopic examination (Chew, 1966).

With no known organic pathology, the cause of hoarseness, like that of harshness, is excessive muscular tension in the laryngeal area. Consistent or prolonged hoarseness may also cause (or be the result of) organic deviation of the laryngeal mechanism, particularly the vocal folds. Such vocal quality is often heard in patients with vocal nodules and contact ulcers. Like harshness, this disorder also has a rough or noisy quality. Moore and Thompson (1965) and others (Yanaghiara, 1964, 1967a, 1967b; Von Leden, 1968) have shown that there are noise components within the fundamental frequency and higher formant ranges that enable listeners to perceive these particular characteristics in the voice. In fact, Von Leden (1968) has been able to recognize at least four types (Type I, II, III, IV) of hoarseness based on various aerodynamic and acoustic measures.

The problem of hoarseness also exists in children. Certainly this is evident, particularly in males, when the voice is changing due to puberty. Many children also exhibit vocal nodules. Baynes (1966) has stated that there are three major causes for hoarseness in children: (1) laryngitis; (2) abuse and misuse of the voice, together with excessive tension; and (3) the mutation period in the male adolescent.

Aphonia (Psychogenic Aphonia, Pseudoparalytic Aphonia, Hysterical Aphonia)

Aphonia, is literally, total loss of the voice. However, in most cases there is whispering; but in extreme cases the whispering is so soft as to make the total speech output unintelligible. This disorder is a fairly well-known (although not common) functional voice disorder occurring most frequently in young girls and women. It has been reported in children and men, but this is rare.

The history usually indicates a very sudden onset. In many cases the individual awakens one morning without voice. There is usually no immediate recognition of any disturbing or disagreeable situation which may have caused the behavior. Deeper investigation may reveal some emotional conflict in family or professional relationships.

During the examination the patient is asked to cough. This will usually be done with a normal sound, indicating that the folds are not paralyzed, although there are some patients who have been examined many times and who have "learned" to cough without voice. However, the non-existence of paralyzed folds is usually confirmed by laryngoscopy, although there are some patients who can make such an examination impossible because of a very strong gag reflex. The diagnosis, as a rule, is not difficult because aphonia will otherwise occur only in gross organic pathology—such as extensive tumor growth, a very large vocal fold polyp, or vocal fold paralysis—which all plainly show visible deviations upon examination. However, there have been some cases of vocal fold paralysis with overlaid functional aphonia.

> Mrs. S., age sixty-seven, was seen for the problem of aphonia. Initial examination revealed a paralyzed cord and was considered the cause of the aphonia. However, during further examinations a normal cough was heard. Continued investigation revealed that she had had a strumectomy fifteen years before and had been talking since then. Through further questioning it was discovered that Mrs. S. was widowed and was recently left completely alone by the marriage of her daughter. Mrs. S. received some assistance through counseling and is presently talking.

The prognosis in cases of aphonia is variable. Sometimes the reaction is of very short duration in a person with a predominantly healthy personality. However, if the conflict is not solved, then the prognosis becomes exceedingly more guarded. Therapy is mainly supportive and cathartic. In some instances physicians have used faradic current or the introduction of glycerine in the larynx to bring about immediate use of the voice. At times this has been successful, but must be used with caution. In long-standing cases a more concentrated program of speech therapy and psychological counseling may be required.

Spastic Dysphonia (Dysphonia Spastica, Vocal Stuttering)

Another disorder of functional origin (although differences do exist in the literature as to the cause) which occurs very rarely is spastic dysphonia. Phonation is characterized by a very strained, shaky, and tense vocal sound. This disorder has been referred to as "vocal stuttering" because of the great strain to phonate and the accompanying tensions evident during phonation. In this type of phonation it appears that the breath stream is at times being locked by a stiffly closed glottis. Also, as is evident at times in stuttering, after several laboriously uttered words a perfectly normal sentence may follow. Spastic dysphonia occurs at least four times more frequently in men than in women. Clinical experience has indicated that these people feel neglected, are having financial difficulties, or have suffered some great personal loss. Psychotherapy has been advocated or a combination of psychotherapy and voice therapy. The prognosis is somewhat guarded and relapses do occur.

The exact cause or causes of this disorder is unknown. There exists in the literature some differences of opinion as to whether the etiology of spastic dysphonia is of psychogenic or organic origin. People such as Heaver (1958), Bloch 1965), and Cornut (1965) all present evidence leading to a psychogenic basis. Robe, et al. (1960) and Aronson, et al. (1968a, 1968b) state that this disorder should be viewed as having an organic basis because of the neurological signs evident in the populations they investigated. Because of our own position that this disorder is predominantly a "learned" behavior, it is included in the present section.

SUMMARY

This chapter has attempted discussion of some functional dysphonias. It has by no means included all such disorders. Problems of mutation (pitch) were discussed in a previous chapter. Although many of the disorders—such as harshness, hoarseness, breathiness, and aphonia—may be related to organic deviations, they have been discussed only in terms of their functional aspects in this section.

Chapter 5

ORGANIC CHANGES OF THE VOCAL FOLD AS A CONSEQUENCE OF DYSFUNCTION

In the previous chapter those voice disorders in which no organic pathology was noted were discussed and referred to as functional dysphonias. It is, however, highly possible that the continued misuse and abuse of the voice, although functional in nature, may eventually lead to organic pathology of the vocal mechanism. Prolonged use of improper vocal habits may cause the vocal mechanism to set a defensive reaction leading to changes of the vocal folds such as nodules, contact ulcers, polyps, edema, and other laryngeal pathologies.

VOCAL NODULES

(Chronic Nodular Laryngitis, Screamer's Nodes)

Vocal nodules are probably the most frequently seen organic voice disorder occurring in adults. Although the statistics of distribution varies, this disorder occurs more frequently in adult females than in adult males (Heaver, 1958). Children also develop nodules, and the incidence is higher than in the adult population.

We are in agreement with both Moore (1971) and Greene (1964) that vocal nodules are always the result of trauma to the vocal folds. This trauma is brought about by overtaxation and misuse of the voice, the origin of which may be habitual dysphonia. In a vibration pattern which deviates from normal there may be points where the energy is not sufficiently dissipated, and it is here where a nodule will arise due to hyperplasia of the epithelium and/or submucous edema. These benign, paired, symmetrical growths are localized thickenings varying in size from small pointed growths to more polyp-like elevations. The typical location of nodules is on the border of the anterior and middle third of the vocal folds. From a histological point of view, a stage of fluid build-up initially occurs. As vocal abuse continues, there appears a vascular invasion followed by a complete fibrous organization which gives birth to a small polyp-like elevation. Luchsinger and Arnold (1965), Ash (1962), and Arnold (1962) fully discuss the pathology, histology, and laryngoscopic appearance of the vocal nodule.

People whose professions require them to speak a great deal are the ones who are most usually seen for diagnosis and treatment of vocal nodules. The complaint of the individual with nodules can date from several weeks to several months. Often these patients complain of a "sore" throat or a "lump" in the throat. With those individuals whose profession requires a great deal of vocalization, it is reported that their throats feel "better" after a "week-end" rest than at the end of the week. Patients also indicate that when they are emotionally upset, their voices become much worse, until in some patients, aphonia results. Almost all patients report using their voices excessively and/or abusing it (continued phonation while suffering laryngitis, colds, etc.).

When the larynx is examined by indirect laryngoscopy the vocal folds appear to be of normal color, with a slight red region around each nodule; the borders of the folds are not straight. On phonation there is incomplete closure in the middle part of the folds. If stroboscopy is utilized, the consistency of the nodules can be more readily observed. Round edematous swellings vibrate in phase with the whole vocal fold. Older, more fibrous elevations can be a hindrance to the vibratory pattern so that only the posterior part of the glottis may be seen to be vibrating. In some instances different vibrational patterns can be seen in the anterior and posterior parts of the vocal folds. The resulting vocal quality is usually breathiness, poor chest resonance and lack of overtones.

Surgical intervention is necessary only when the nodes are large and fibrous and have been present for a prolonged period of time. Removal is done by direct laryngoscopy. However, in most cases, voice therapy is the treatment of choice. In many cases, voice rest is prescribed. When the prescription calls for absolute speechlessness for a long period of time, the nodules can, if voice rest is followed rigorously, be reduced or completely disappear. The question is, however, what will happen following the resumption of vocalization? If the patient continues to maintain his faulty habits of phonation, the disorder will recur. Vocal rest, therefore, should not be the *only* treatment, except, perhaps, in situations where there is a brief period of over-taxation of the voice (such as politicians during a vigorous campaign). Voice therapy is indicated in most patients. This would consist generally of exercises to improve respiratory control and to maintain the proper balance and tension of the laryngeal structure.

The vocal nodules of children are much different. They are also benign epithelian reactions, but these give rise to spindle-like thickenings on both vocal folds. These are by no means as fibrous as the nodules seen in adults. Surgical treatment of children with nodules is never done. Brodnitz (1965) states:

> The screamer's nodules of children should be left strictly alone, since they respond very well to improvement in vocal habits and to the simpler forms of voice training. Even children of early school age can be taught to handle their voices with some care, to avoid the worst forms of vocal abuse, and to practice types of vocal exercises that can be presented as a kind of game.

Wilson (1961, 1962) presents a system of therapeutic procedures for children and adolescents with vocal nodules.

POLYPS

A vocal cord polyp may develop from edematous folds when the effusion is concentrated in one place and where it pushes the epithelium forward. Polyps may occur along the whole membraneous part of the vocal fold. However, like the nodule (which is a member of the polyp family) they tend to be seen in the anterior and middle third of the fold. They are unilateral and vary greatly in size and shape. "They may be pedunculated, projecting into the glottis, or they may hang down and become difficult to visualize" (Brodnitz, 1958). While it has been generally thought that a vocal fold polyp is the result of abuse and misuse of the voice, it often occurs without evidence of such origin. It would seem then that even without vocal abuse, a polyp can, because of its interference with the normal mode of vocal fold vibration, be the cause of a voice quality disorder.

Laryngoscopic examination of the polyp is not always easy or revealing. Because of its particular location on the folds near the anterior commissure, it may be hidden from sight by an overhanging epiglottis. Another misleading factor is that the polyp may be hidden under the folds during phonation. However, stroboscopic examination will aid greatly in determining its presence or absence. In an individual with vocal polyps, the quality of the voice may change from moment to moment, from very harsh to near normal, depending on whether the polyp is interfering with the vibrational pattern. In most instances, vocal polyps must be removed surgically, and when incorrect use of the voice exists, voice therapy must follow as soon as it is advisable. A polyp of the vocal cord will never be absorbed. There are some instances in which they have become necrotic and have been coughed up involuntarily, or sponaneously cured when a very young polyp ruptures and its contents run off.

VOCAL FOLD EDEMA

Vocal fold edema is essentially a swelling of the vocal folds. The epithelium which covers the muscles and the ligament of the vocal fold is attached to the underlying tissues by a loose connective tissue. The space between the vocal fold and this epithelial layer is called the subepithelial space of Reinke. Accumulation of tissue fluid in this space is called vocal fold edema.

Vocal fold edema occurs symmetrically. It can be a complication of acute laryngitis, particularly if the voice has been abused or misused during laryngitis; it may also be due to overtaxation of the vocal organs. An allergic condition may give rise to swelling of the aryepiglottic folds, but never of the vocal folds. Edema of one vocal fold may develop in a glottis which does not close completely, as in the case of lateral fixation where the edema is primarily a compensatory effort. This is a rare occurrence.

During laryngoscopic examination the rosy or pallid, glossy appearance of the edematous folds cannot fail to be recognized. It is of greater diagnostic difficulty to recognize a slight degree of vocal fold edema. Evaluation of the vocal function will reveal that the vocal range is extended a few semitones downward, and falsetto tones are difficult, or even impossible, to produce. Because of the suppleness (pliability) of the vocal folds due to subepithelial fluid, the voice in the patient with edema is of a low frequency and has an exaggerated chest resonance. The vibration rate can be 80 Hz and lower. This low rate of vibration approaches the vocal fry sound.

Light and moderate degrees of vocal fold edema can recover with voice rest and voice therapy. The prognosis is dependent upon the time necessary for the colloidal mass under the epithelium to be reabsorbed, which may take months. In more severe cases, however, incision and drainage or removal of the swollen mucosa is indicated. The folds, which are stripped of their swollen epithelium, will be overgrown with healthy epithelium. The stripping has to be done on one vocal fold at a time, in two tempi, with ten to fourteen days between, during which time only quiet whispering is allowed.

CONTACT ULCER

In 1928, Chevalier Jackson (1928) described this disorder, and in fact coined the term "contact ulcer." Although Jackson is credited with the identification, Peacher (1947) gave the best description of contact ulcers when she stated:

> On direct laryngoscopy, a tiny point denoting ulcer is seen on the edge, involving the almost perpendicular surface of the arytenoid cartilage. The lesion is exposed to view during respiration but on phonation its internal surface is in contact with the internal surface of the opposite arytenoid eminence which may or may not be

> ulcerated. The bordering mucosa is inflamed. Sometimes the edges of the ulcer are the same color as the surrounding mucosa. Granulomas formed from the granulation material are sometimes seen in the bed of the ulcer though, in most cases, it is only epithelialized. . . . Grossly, the tissue is a mass of about 2-8 mm.

The lesions are usually located at the dorsal end of the vocal cords at their attachment to the vocal process of the arytenoid cartilage. "Unlike vocal nodules they are indentations rather than projections . . ." (Van Riper and Irwin, 1958). In Europe this condition is known under the name pachydermia of the larynx (Brodnitz, 1961).

Contact ulcers are very common. Jackson (1935) reports treating 127 cases in forty years, Baker (1954) observed nineteen cases in sixteen years, and Brodnitz (1961) treated twenty-six cases in a period of eight years. This disorder seems to be associated with middle age. Peacher (1947) reported that the average of the sample she studied was fifty years old. Brodnitz (1961) confirms this and states that the age range of his patients was forty to fifty-five years. This disorder is seen more often in males than in females. Peacher (1947) reports a 15 to 1 ratio.

The consensus is that contact ulcers are caused by vocal abuse, particularly when the individual puts forth a great deal of effort in attempting to speak at a pitch level that is too low. However, many interesting postulations have been set forth in an attempt to establish additional etiologies for this abnormality. Peacher (1947) states that "occupation seems to have a definite etiologic bearing on the condition." There is a high incidence of contact ulcers in individuals whose work requires a great deal of talking. Brodnitz (1961) found that those with the most contact ulcers were business executives whose work involved a great deal of speaking.

Tobacco and alcohol have been mentioned as possible factors in the production of contact ulcers. Jackson (1935) and Peroni (1933) talk of infected tonsils and chronic suppurative disease of the nasal accessory sinuses as probable causes. Moses (1954) states that contact ulcers develop under emotional stress. Peacher (1947) considers a contact ulcer "a disorder of function produced by defective action of the larynx which is referred to as misuse of the voice." In other words, the primary cause of contact ulcer is voice abuse.

The chief vocal symptom of contact ulcer is hoarseness. These patients also exhibit tension, particularly of the speech musculature. Speech is initiated with a hard glottal attack and the voice pitch is noticeably low. The voice tires easily and the individual complains of a constant need to clear his throat. Pitch variability is also greatly restricted.

There is agreement that in treating contact ulcers, vocal reeducation is necessary. Some authorities strongly recommend vocal rest, but such a prescription without vocal reeducation can be considered as only a temporary cure for contact ulcers. If the disorders have existed for a considerable period of time and a significant period of vocal rest has not been successful in reducing the ulceration and granulation, then the lesion must be surgically excised. However, as previously mentioned, vocal reeducation is essential in the management of contact ulcers regardless of the medical treatment involved.

CHRONIC LARYNGITIS, KERATOSIS, LEUKOPLAKIA

There is general agreement that chronic laryngitis can be the result of vocal abuse alone, although other vocal irritants can bring about this disorder (Greene, 1964; Myerson, 1964; Moore, 1971; and Boone, 1971). However, there are differences of opinion as to whether or not the hyperplastic forms of chronic laryngitis, keratosis, and leukoplakia are due primarily to vocal abuse. Boone (1971) states that keratosis and leukoplakia are not the result of vocal abuse or misuse. Greene (1964) issues no statement regarding the etiological factors relating to these disorders, but discusses them in her chapter dealing with vocal abuse. Myerson (1964), in his discussion of these three disorders, states "It is customary to impugn smoking, vocal abuse, various forms of irritation, chronic inflammation and vitamin deficiency, when considering etiology." Since these differences do exist it is felt that chronic laryngitis, keratosis, and leukoplakia can be considered within this section.

Chronic Laryngitis

The diagnosis of chronic laryngitis is based on the findings of a laryngoscopic examination of the vocal folds: the larynx mucosa is red; the vocal folds show a thickening, reddish appearance and an irregular surface; ropy secretions and fibrous exudate can cover the surface of the fold. Chronic laryngitis can be discerned from other local deviations by its diffuse appearance. Brodnitz (1965) refers to two types of chronic laryngitis. He states that the laryngoscopic picture in both forms is identical and "The diagnosis of nonspecific laryngitis can be made only if all possible sources of infection or irritation can be excluded— such as allergies, chemical irritation, abuse of nicotine and/or alcohol—and if vocal abuse can be established." The major vocal symptoms are hoarseness, limited tonal range, and pitch breaks.

In principle, this disorder is reversible. This means the epithelium will return to normal if all causal factors are eliminated. The first step in treatment is an attempt to alleviate medically any disease of internal and/or otorhinolaryngological nature that may tend to aggravate the situation. It has been noted that chronic laryngitis reacts well to vocal rest, although voice therapy is strongly advocated.

Keratosis, Leukoplakia

Common to these disorders is a strong reaction of the epithelium (inflammation, thickening, hyperplasia) and that they occur mainly in men. These are benign growths usually localized on the anterior halves of the vocal folds. The history of patients with these disorders indicates the presence of a rather constant and consistent hoarseness over a long period of time, with complaints of easy fatigue of the voice, dry throat, difficulties with swallowing, and "tough" secretions. Leukoplakia can be a prodromal stage of vocal fold carcinoma. In all instances primary treatment is medical, followed by voice therapy.

SUMMARY

It appears evident from the previous discussion that functional dysphonia, vocal abuse, can result in organic changes of the vocal folds. These changes not only further complicate and distort phonation but may also cause various degrees of physical discomfort. Such organic changes resulting from a functional etiology further indicate the need fo greater cooperation between the laryngologist and the speech pathologist, since in most instances any medical treatment should be followed up by voice therapy if the patient is to benefit fully.

Chapter 6

THERAPY

IN ADDITION TO specific treatment suggested for the various disorders, there are also methods of treatment with a general and broad area of indication. Voice disorders, whether of predominantly organic or functional nature, can be treated in varying degrees in a similar fashion.

Therapy attempts to obtain the best adaptation for optimal phonation to the given anatomical situation. In order to achieve this goal the therapist must be concerned with breath control, relaxation, and vocal exercises. Although these are presented as separate entities in the discussion, the therapeutic process must be approached as a total system. In other words, breathing, relaxation, and vocal exercises have a complex interaction with each other and cannot be treated separately.

BREATH CONTROL

The concept of the importance of breath control and faulty breathing, as related to voice disorders, in the past has been greatly overplayed. Presently, little emphasis has been devoted to faulty respiration and its role in maintenance of vocal disorders. Both points of view are extreme. There are many individuals with voice disorders who are not able to control their breathing movements adequately because they occur partly automatically and partly voluntarily. In other words, the control of respiration occupies a place between the voluntarily controlled movements of the head, trunk, and extremities, and automatically controlled movements such as those of the heart and the digestive tract.

During respiration, the diaphragm, in the inspiration phase, moves downward and forward, thereby exerting pressure on the abdominal contents. This causes an enlargement of the thoracic cavity as well as outward or forward movement of the abdominal wall. When the muscle fibers are relaxed the diaphragm moves upward, the thoracic cavity decreases, and the abdominal wall moves inward on the expiration phase of the respiratory cycle. This is the type of respiratory pattern noted in a condition of rest or relaxation.

Some individuals with voice disorders may have related deficiencies in breath control and, therefore, utilize faulty breathing patterns. One of the most common has been referred to as chest breathing or high thoracic breathing. The utilization of

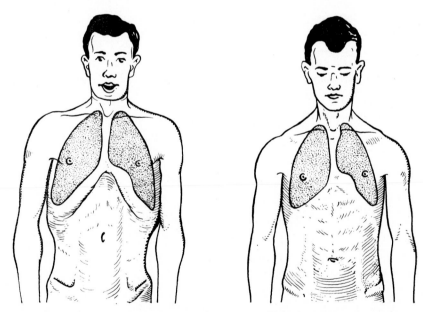

Figure 7. Paradox or inverse breathing movement. Left after inspiration; right: after expiration. The diaphragm is drawn upward during the movement for inspiration as can be seen from the inward movement of the abdominal wall. Normally the diaphragm moves downward and the abdominal wall outward on inspiration. "From: De pathologische stembandfunctie Stafleu, Leiden Neth."

such a breathing pattern is an inefficient way of displacing air. Those individuals who use such a pattern tend to exhibit tension and anxiety.

Disturbed breathing and insufficient breath control disrupt the delicate balance needed to produce the desired sound. This is evidenced by alterations in posture, body movement, breathing pattern, and voice during situations involving emotional tension. Such deviations tend to make more difficult the maintenance of proper breath support for the production of adequate vocal quality. (Luchsinger and Arnold [1966] and Vennard [1962] thoroughly discuss the concept of breath support.)

Another concept related to breath control has been that of proper posture. Moore (1971) states, ". . . it is unlikely that poor posture in itself causes voice disorders, but it is an important element in voice therapy." In the words of Martienssen-Lohman:

> The singer assumes a posture and a form of complete breathing with assured rest in the upper part of the trunk and allows only the lower part of the trunk to move. The posture is such that the quiet and wide attitude of the upper part can be sustained for long periods of time. A position which the old Italian masters used to indicate to their pupils "come una statua" (1956).

In this posture of elongated spine, wide thorax, and low diaphragm, the conditions of optimal phonation are present.

RELAXATION

The healthy, relaxed state of the organism may be called "eutonia": possessing the right degree of tension for the situation and ready to adapt this at any moment. Moore (1957) says, "relaxation is a dynamic balance, in which the opposing groups of muscles exert just enough reciprocating tension upon each other to accomplish the desired movement with perfect control."

The section indicates that states of anxiety and tension are sometimes associated with voice disorders. Boone (1971) feels that most problems of dysphonia result from hyperfunction and hypertonia, and therapeutic programs involving general body relaxation are useful. In dealing with various dysphonias, the clinician is often confronted with patients who find it difficult to relax. "Tension and vocal strain are recognized by pathologists as causes of numerous vocal difficulties. It is easier to achieve efficient, effective voice production if you can relax your entire body to a level of tension just adequate to the job at hand" (Hanley and Thurman, 1963).

Methods for relaxation training have been described by Jacobson (1934), Alexander (1955), and others. Relaxation exercises may, in themselves, relieve some psychological anxieties or tensions of the individual; however, a more "psychotherapeutic" approach may be necessary. Relaxation should be applied in a systematic desensitization program. The steps chosen should be small enough so that they are always within reach of the patient. Even when the patient has good insight of his own inadequate functioning he is unable to extinguish his previously learned behavior. The goal of relaxation therapy is to attain more adequate functioning of the organism and more adequate reaction and attitudes in the environment.

VOCAL EXERCISES

Relaxation and breath control exercises can be carried out simultaneously with phonation exercises. Indeed, establishing a feeling for the right posture and movement should also go hand in hand with the identification of the optimal sound quality. In this instance, vocal exercises do not refer to "exercises" of the muscles of the larynx, but rather to the total interplay of breath control, relaxation and phonation. (Perhaps the term *practice* as suggested by Brodnitz [1965] should be used rather than exercise.)

A system incorporating the simultaneous use of breath control, relaxation, and phonation has been suggested by Svend Smith of Copenhagen, Denmark. This method has never been formally published, although it is widely used in, and taught to, European logopedists through seminars in various countries. (Smith also uses his "accent-method" in the treatment of stutterers in order to reestablish the normal rhythmical stress patterns of fluent speech.) The basics of the method, as presented here, may reflect some of the biases (that is—a subjective interpretation) of the authors and, therefore, may not be truly representative of the original thinking of Smith.

This therapeutic approach is based on the principle of automatic regulation. Smith feels that voice production involves more than laryngeal structures. He considers total body movement and its effect on body position, good breath control, and tension factors with the premise that optimal conditions in these areas will result in normal voice production. He is concerned with the rhythm of breathing and the rhythmical control of body movements and attempts to bring the body into a state of "relaxed readiness." This is accomplished by having the patient imitate, in a rhythmic pattern, the movements of the clinician. The rhythmic movement reduces tension and aids the patient in achieving a balanced state in the concerned musculature.

The patient is shown that the abdominal wall moves outward on inspiration and then inward on expiration. The clinician will demonstrate, then have the patient participate, continuing in a rhythmical alternating fashion; that is, when the clinician is active, the patient is passive.

When this rhythmic form of breathing is acquired (which usualy can be accomplished very early in the session) phonation is introduced. Phonation is started with a very soft, breathy sound, and on expiration a vowel is produced. As this phase proceeds the vocal rhythmical forms become longer and the accents can be changed. The pitch may vary with the accents. Smith feels that the correct pitch for the individual will come about during the process of the exercises when the improperly used stress positions are reduced. Therefore, there is no need for the patient to imitate the pitch patterns of the clinician.

When adequate breathing-voice coordination has been achieved with both soft, breathy sounds and loud, nonbreathy sounds, vocalizations utilizing consonant-vowel articulation is introduced and further exercises with nonsense syllables is started. Such a program is expected to be carried on in the home environment, with the use of a tape recorder, in conjunction with the clinical program.

It is this rhythmical pattern, with accompanying bodily movement—first in breathing, then phonation—that is the nucleus of the Smith method. Though this tension is reduced and aspects of relaxation, breathing and voice exercises are improved without undue therapeutic attention to each area separately. The Smith approach neither lends itself easily, nor is done justice by, written "instructionalization." Considerable observation and practice are indicated both for therapist, who must become thoroughly familiar and at ease with the methodology, and for the patient, who must engage in very active participation (Lerman, 1972).

STRUCTURING THERAPY

In voice therapy, the vocal disorder is not treated as an entity in and of itself, but rather the individual with the disorder is treated. It is not possible to separate one from the other. A good clinician does not base a therapeutic program on the name of the disease, but rather on the specific needs of the individual with the voice dysfunction.

It is fairly well-known that individuals with vocal dysfunction are highly resistant to change. Although they may produce adequate voice quality within the clinical situation, the majority are apt to revert to their old vocal habits in situations outside of the clinical realm. It would be worthless then if voice therapy were limited only to the clinical situation. Any efficacious voice treatment must gradually introduce everyday life situations into therapy. If voice is learned, then vocal dysfunction (in the case of habitual dysphonia and perhaps in some organic cases) must be approached as a conditioned response to the discriminative stimuli and consequences of everyday life. A program of applied behavior analysis in which the faulty pattern is changed and the more adequate pattern is then maintained would be applicable here.

Learning theories have revealed two principles that can be, and are, utilized in the therapeutic process: successive approximation (shaping) and stimulus generalization. In successive approximation the old patterns are gradually, in a step-by-step process, replaced by the more desired behavior. There is no systematic way of approaching this process; it might simply be said that the "measuring" of the steps is the art of the clinician. Stimulus generalization means that the new behavior, if practiced regularly within and without the clinical situation, will continue to occur in situations similar to those encountered during practice.

Although it has been stated previously that the therapeutic program should be geared to the individual and not to the disorder, there are certain premises on which most therapy for voice disorders can be based.

1. A relationship must be established in which the patient can view the clinician not only as an expert, but as a person whom he can respect and a person whom he feels will be understanding and able to assist him when he has to cope with the radical modification of his habitual reactions and attitudes. These individuals are resistant to change, not only in their vocal habits, but in their attitudes and feelings regarding the disorder as well. The relationship must be a positively reinforcing one.

2. The patient and clinician must both be aware of the behavior they desire to change. What is the patient doing to produce this undesirable sound? What is the difference between this and a more desirable vocal quality? The patient must realize that it is *his* misuse and abuse of the voice that is causing the disorder. Certainly in those oragnic disorders in which there has been permanent alteration of the mechanism, the patient should be aware that through some compensatory effort more suitable and acceptable phonation can be achieved.

3. A more suitable voice quality must be targeted. The range of voice possibilities of the patient is scanned by means of breathing and voice practice (Smith method), and the best production is then reinforced. The clinician himself does not serve as a model, but rather the desired vocal behavior is found within the patient's own repertoire. The achievement of a more suitable voice production during this "scanning" period is continuously reinforced as a motivating force for the patient.

4. When a satisfactory vocal quality is achieved in the therapy session, a program should be designed whereby this desired behavior will be able to occur at its maximum and be continually, positively reinforced.

5. In order for the new behavior to be maintained, the patient must practice regularly and frequently outside of the clinical situation. It is suggested that when the clinician is sure that the patient can produce the desired vocal quality at will and with ease, the patient be placed on a regime of five minutes of practice every hour.

6. If the patient continues to participate in therapy in this manner, then the phase of morphological adaptation will take place. In other words, the secondary organic changes, such as chronic nodular laryngitis, tend to disappear and the organic structure returns to its former healthy state.

The initial part of this program (Steps 1 through 4) can be achieved early in the therapeutic process. The latter phases (Steps 5 and 6) may take several weeks or even months. Experience has shown that when utilizing this systematic approach (in conjunction with the Smith method), frequent and active therapy is the most efficient and effective way to achieve success with any given individual.

Additional Therapy: Medical Aspects

A frequent complaint in voice disorders is excessive phlegm, which is felt as an impediment to phonation. It may occur as a result of bronchitis or tracheitis following a cold. Also, misuse of the voice, when the folds do not close and do not vibrate with full amplitude, can retard the normal movement of bronchial secretions through the glottis. The symptom is then reinforced by its own consequences. What occurs is frequent rasping and coughing, which in turn is more harmful to the vocal folds. Various drugs can be prescribed for drying up excess secretion and for stimulating serous secretion. At times it is necessary to use drugs that depress coughing reactions. When codeine is applied at the right moment, vocal fold edema may be prevented as a result of a severe cough. The direct application of drugs on the epithelium of the folds is seldom indicated. Etching substances may have untold consequences. States of depression or anxiety have to be treated by appropriate measures. Drugs may be of benefit in these cases. There have been reported instances in which vocal nodules in children have been seen to disappear under the sole effect of sedatives. However, one has to be sure that the cure is not worse than the illness.

Chapter 7

PRIMARY ORGANIC DYSPHONIA

ORGANIC ANOMALIES or defects of the laryngeal mechanism are seldom the primary causes of a voice disorder. Generally, the greatest number of voice disorders are functional in nature, although there may be some with secondary organic changes. However, there are certain organic voice disorders which occur with enough frequency to be considered in this chapter.

LARYNGEAL PARALYSIS

Paralysis of the vocal folds can result from many causes. Such a paralysis is always more than just a dysfunction of the voice-producing mechanism. It can be a sign of a serious central nervous system lesion. However, there are indications that the greatest percentage of cases of vocal fold paralysis have resulted from damage to the recurrent laryngeal nerve, a branch of the tenth cranial nerve, Vagus, during an operation on the thyroid gland. In a study by Clerf (1953), fifty-nine of sixty-eight patients with unilateral paralysis were reported to have occurred after thyroidectomy. Since there is a higher incidence of thyroidectomy in women than men, it follows that vocal fold paralysis is more prevalent in females.

There are other causes by which innervation of the larynx can be disrupted: (1) tumors and toxic nerve reactions in the region of the larynx, the pharynx, and the thorax. This is especially true on the left side because of the longer trajectory, of the left recurrent laryngeal nerve coursing around the aortic arch. These tumors may be compressing the vagus nerve. (2) Lesions in the area of the nucleus of the vagus nerve (bulbar paralysis). Generally speaking, however, the cause in a large number of cases remains unknown. Landman (1966), in a study of recurrent laryngeal paralysis, listed unknown causes for almost one third of his cases.

The individual who may be suffering from laryngeal paralysis might complain of a weak voice or aphonia or difficulty in breathing. If there is no history of a recent thyroid operation, then the diagnostic information must concern itself with recent illnesses such as measles, encephalitis, viral infections, and with signs such as difficulties with swallowing, increasing hoarseness, onset of slight hypernasality, etc. It is vital that the diagnostician make every attempt to determine the etiological factors involved in the paralysis because such symptoms may be indicative of some CNS lesions. The earlier the diagnosis, the more chance for a favorable prognosis.

The diagnosis of laryngeal paralysis is made primarily via the laryngoscopic examination, as well as inspection and palpation of the areas of the neck. Stroboscopy should be part of the laryngoscopic examination. This method allows for a more discriminating diagnosis and enables the laryngologist to determine whether or not a disorder is of psychogenic nature.

The symptoms presented during stroboscopic examination of the vocal folds will vary depending on the extent of damage to the nerve supply of the larynx and whether the paralysis is uni- or bilateral. In a unilateral paralysis, a hypotonia on the affected side can be observed during stroboscopy, and the amplitude of vibration of the affected cord is larger than that of the unaffected cord. When the glottis is not closed completely, the paralyzed cord may be seen to vibrate in an irregular fashion. Buch (1972) states:

> The paralyzed vocal lip rapidly becomes hollowed out or atrophied and later a change also appears in the position of the Arytenoid cartilage. The glottis becomes twisted and a certain compensation in the movements of the healthy vocal lip appears to set in. With stroboscopy, the abnormal oscillation pattern is seen with predominence of the vertical movement. This is important, in diagnosing the difference from the phenomenon, Ary-fixation.

The effect on vocal function, as noted during the examination, is dependent upon the position of the vocal folds in paralysis. Clinical experience indicates that in most cases of such laryngeal paralysis, vocal function has been affected, varying from mild to severe. In a bilateral paralysis, with the cords in the median or para-median position, there is usually adequate vocal quality; however, there may be some respiratory difficulty. If the glottal opening is too wide, there will be more air used during speech with subsequent poor vocal quality and sensations such as dizziness, headaches, and possibly the hyperventilation syndrome.

In all likelihood the speech pathologist will be more concerned with the individual with a unilateral paralysis. Once again, the effect on the voice is dependent upon the position of the paralyzed cord. In a progressive paralysis, according to the *Law of Semon-Rosenbach,* the affected vocal cord would begin in the median position and later move to the intermedian position. In practice, the reverse is now usually seen: the paralyzed cord, initially in the intermedian position, later moves towards the median position. As a consequence, the voice of the patient improves gradually. Also, the healthy cord can, by practice, compensate for the lack of movement in the paralyzed cord. When the paralyzed cord is in the paramedian position, the healthy cord can effect adequate closure by crossing the midline, and voice quality may not be disturbed. If the cord is paralyzed in a more lateral or intermedian position, the healthy cord cannot compensate and the vocal quality will be breathy, weak, lacking in chest register, and have a greatly reduced range.

Decursus is determined by: (1) the degree of progression of the paralysis, (2) the degree of reinnervation, and (3) the degree of compensation by the muscles which are not paralyzed and which can partly restore function.

THERAPY

Therapy depends upon several factors: (1) the type of paralysis, (2) the length of time the paralysis has been in existence, (3) the course that the paralysis is expected to take, and (4) the motivation of the individual.

In the case of a unilateral paralysis in the para- or inter-median position, it will be necessary to improve glottal closure. Several methods have been employed to achieve this closure. Many individuals have suggested voice training with the purpose of utilizing the healthy aspects of the laryngeal mechanism to compensate for the paralysis and to retain as much of the inner-vation which may still exist.

> Recently a college professor with vocal fold fixation of unknown origin was treated with voice therapy. Therapy consisted of vocal exercises and vigorous expiration thrusts and simultaneous vigorous movements with the arms and shoulders, the so-called "thrust exercises," which stimulate glottal constriction. Although he re-gained a near normal voice, he also had some very visible and obvious compensatory neck muscle activity.

In a therapeutic approach of this type, care must be taken that such compensatory muscle movement does not become dis-tracting or even harmful. However, some patients who have not received voice therapy have developed such a system on their own.

In the recent past some physicians have suggested that muscle tonus could be maintained by means of regular galvanic or faradic stimulation. Theoretically, it is very doubtful that this type of treatment is of any assistance. Its application, however, has been widely accepted among phoniatrists who feel it should at least be combined with voice therapy. Brodnitz (1965) states: "In the early stages of treatment, the effect of faradization is probably largely psychological but its use is justified because it reassures the patient that something is being done, outside of exercises. Once phonation is re-established, faradization is useful in strengthening vocal intensity and increasing range." Such an approach should not be undertaken by the speech pathologist without medical assistance.

If the paralysis is one of long-standing, a year or more, and the functioning cord is unable to make the necessary compen-satory movement to achieve approximation, the displacement of the paralyzed cord to a more median position should be considered. This can be accomplished by injection of an artificial substance. A suspension of Teflon® in a viscous base has been used and seems to be most suitable. It appears to be an easy matter to inject, and research seems to indicate that there is little danger of undesired tissue reaction. The literature in this area is very extensive, and for information concerning the criteria for the utilization of Teflon and its advantages and disadvantages, the reader is referred to Arnold (1964), Kirchner, et al. (1966), von Leden, et al. (1967), and Robin (1965a, 1965b). Rubin (1966) has also made an excellent film on Teflon injection.

When voice therapy for a unilateral paralysis in the paramedian position is instituted, the goal is for the development of adequate phonation in relation to the organic deviation. Perhaps a short waiting period after the discovery of the paralysis is needed before therapy begins, as there is the possibility that a vocal fold paralysis in the paramedian position may eventually change to an even more median position. If this does occur, it is difficult to determine if this is caused by a partial reinnervation (causing the adduction effect of the cricothyroid muscle to enter into play) or by compensatory activity of other muscles that are not affected by paralysis. Faaborg-Anderson (1964), in his discussion of the position of paretic vocal cords, states:

> . . . I am convinced that the position of the vocal cord is affected differently by partial and total paresis. In many cases of immovable vocal cord, it can be demonstrated electromyographically that there is only a partial paresis as several motor units are still functioning, though fewer than normally. In fact, to my mind, it is surprisingly seldom that abrogated electric activity or total denervation of the intrinsic larynx muscles are found in cases of immovable cords.
>
> I believe this may influence the position of the paretic vocal cord. If a certain number of motor units are still functioning, the muscles will have a certain "tension," although they may not be able to contract actively. In the majority of cases, this "tension distribution" will probably follow certain laws which will produce a characteristic position of the paretic vocal cord, but it is conceivable that the "tension distribution" between the different muscles, depending on the kind of lesion involved, in some cases might differ from the norm and thus affect the position of the paretic cord.

Greene (1964) discusses eight types of laryngeal paralysis. However, whether or not voice therapy is instituted depends upon the type and extent of the paralysis, the total organic implication (a symptom of a more serious central nervous system lesion), and further medical intervention.

VOICE DISTURBANCES DUE TO ENDOCRINE DYSFUNCTIONS

The endocrine system regulates many functions of the human organism. Any imbalance or malfunctioning of this system can have a direct effect on phonation. Basically, the pituitary gland, the thyroid and parathyroids, the adrenals, the gonads (testes and ovaries), the islands in the pancreas, and the thymus make up the endocrine system. Each of the hormones produced by these parts is carried through the bloodstream to its specific target tissue or effector organ.

Disturbances in endocrinological functioning may manifest itself in abnormal sexual development and disruption in the normal growth pattern of the larynx and vocal folds. It should be noted, however, that voice abnormalities observed in boys and men after mutation are, as a rule, not the consequence of a deviation in the endocrine system. They occur in the course of a normal functioning endocrine system and are considered and treated as functional disorders (Chapter 3). Insofar as a voice disorder is etiologically linked to a constitutional or acquired deviation or dysfunction of the endocrine system, it is labelled a voice disorder due to endocrine dysfunction.

Hypogonadism (Eunochoidism)

When the hypophysis, an internal secreting gland situated at the base of the brain, secretes few gonadotropines, the consequence is that the gonads produce little testosteron (male hormone relating to the organs of sex and secondary sex characteristics). A small testosteron production can also be due to primary testicular insufficiency, such as seen in Klinefelter's syndrome or in testicular atrophy after mumps. Regardless of the basic cause, if this occurs prior to puberty, secondary sex characteristics do not develop. There will be no hair growth on the face or in the pubic and armpit areas. The body seems to take on a more feminine appearance due to the development of extra fatty tissue on the breasts and the hip area. Laryngeal growth is retarded and the fundamental frequency of the voice remains high.

The individual exhibiting the syndrome of hypogonadism or eunochoidism generally presents the same vocal symptomatology as the castrate, however, to a lesser degree. Castration is an irreversible condition, whereas medication may have some affect on hypogonadism or eunochoidism. Castration of young boys was practiced in the eighteenth and nineteenth centuries by a complete removal of the testicles or ligature of the testicular vessels prior to puberty. The prime reason for this solecistic act was merely for the preservation of the high voice pitch of the young male child. These boys received an intense musical and singing education. The effect of the castrate voice was that these individuals could use adult respiratory and resonance faculties to produce a rather high voice without any particular undue effort (Luchsinger and Arnold, 1965; Moses, 1960).

There should not be any confusion between the voice of the individual with mutation falsetto and that of the patient with hypogonadism or eunuchoidism. The mutation falsetto voice is being produced by an individual with a laryngeal mechanism that has developed normally and has not been affected by an endocrine disturbance. In most cases an adequate laryngoscopic examination will reveal the differences. In cases of doubt, the diagnosis can be corroborated by endocrinological and radiological examinations.

The therapy for hypogonadism is primarily medical. If the examination of the vocal disturbance reveals that the etiology is due to endocrine dysfunction a hormonal substitution therapy with testosteron or gonadotropin is indicated. In most cases such therapy has been successful in restoring some male sexual characteristics and laryngeal growth so that voice therapy may not be necessary.

Virilization of Voice in Women

The voice deviations which have been discussed in Chapter 3 are failures of males to adapt to changes in the normal growth of the laryngeal structures. In women this occurs to a lesser degree. Although there is laryngeal growth in women, it is certainly not to the extent observed in the male, and it does not usually produce a drastic transition to a totally different vocal register. The critical period for the female voice comes much later, in the post-menopause, when the periodic ovulations and menstruations have ceased. A new hormonal balance is established that goes with changes in somatic relations. The elastic tension of the tissues decreases and the epithelium is inclined to atrophy (Damsté, 1964a, 1964b, 1967; Berendes, 1968; and Bauer, 1968).

Our knowledge of the natural development of the female voice in menopause is limited. However, according to F. Martienssen-Lohman (1956), every woman, as she reaches a certain point in her maturity, is threatened with a sort of voice change that occurs in males in puberty. In part, this change may be due to treatment with medication containing anabolic substances which sometimes present side effects and encourage the development of male sex characteristics. These hormones, which have a considerable effect on the protein metabolism and the formation of muscular and connective tissue, are sometimes given for growth problems as early as childhood. Similar types of hormone therapy have been applied to women during periods of convalescense because of after effects of a serious illness. The most extensive utilization of androgenous compounds is for women with climacteric complaints.

Some evidence (Damsté, 1964a, 1964b) suggests that in almost all instances the vocal apparatus undergoes a slight structural change for which there can be compensation to a certain point. However, because of the physiologic aging process there comes a time when these insults cannot be compensated for. The number of women receiving such androgenous substances (usually testosteron preparations) has greatly increased. The individual's sensitivity for such substances, as to the effect on the voice, varies widely. Some women notice a change in voice after only two injections, others after several months of oral therapy. Still others do not complain even if they have suffered profound changes in vocal quality.

The exogenous or more likely iatrogenous causes of virilization in women are much more frequently encountered than the endogenous causes, such as tumors of the ovary and the Stein-Leventhal syndrome. Generally in these endogenous cases, hirsutism is the initial symptom of virilization.

The very early changes in vocal quality, due to virilization, are seldom noticed. Because the change is usually gradual, the patient is not aware of differences until the vocal quality begins to disturb her or call attention to itself. The physician may be even less aware of the side effects of the androgenous or anabolic therapy because he (1) does not know what the side effects are, or (2) associates virilism of the voice with a deep male voice sound, although the early vocal symptomotology does not resemble the adult male voice. Several patients who had made careful self-observation reported that their voices initially "seemed strange," and they found themselves unable to control their singing especially in the higher ranges. They also reported that speaking fatigued them.

When there is laryngeal change due to virilization, there are deviations in quality as well as in pitch. The patient makes a self-diagnosis of "hoarseness," meaning that the timbre is unstable and the voice cracks. The vocal range is not generally decreased, but merely extended into the low tones. In many instances it has been noted that although the higher tones are present, they are unstable and the patient may have some difficult not only in producing but also in sustaining them.

The diagnosis of a vocal dysfunction due to virilization is usually evident from the history, the sound of the voice, and the laryngoscopic finding, although it has sometimes been confused with the beginnings of laryngeal paresis or vocal fold edema. The laryngoscopic image often shows incomplete closure of the dorsal part of the glottis which is remarkably similar to the laryngoscopic picture seen in boys during mutation and has been referred to as the "mutation triangle." This is partially a voluntary hypofunction, the purpose being to avoid the cracking of the voice. The folds may also appear darker in color, yellowish, or grayish, rather than white. Sometimes slightly dilated vessels are seen.

Treatment of virilization of the female voice is very limited. Medically, the application of estrogenic substances (female hormone) has been attempted, but has not proven to be of value. It would appear, then, that there is a permanent change of the connective tissues of the vocal folds due to the androgenous effect of medication. One can only make assumptions, but there may be decreased elastic tension of the conus elasticus and the vocal ligaments. This is an "irreversible" organic situation requiring a new functional approach. Martienssen-Lohman has pointed out that virilization of the voice in a female professional singer may find her career threatened; however, with proper knowledge of what is occurring and by daily exercise of the mixed mid-register in mezzo voice, she may "continue to retain her feminine voice for an indefinite period of time." This mixing of the registers is probably the most important aspect that has to be exercised. The pitch of the speaking voice may be somewhat lower than previously, but this is unavoidable. It is most important that the voice be used in mid-register without inconsistently dropping into chest register. Moore (1971) feels that therapy for this deviant voice quality can best be directed toward "the emphasis of female speech patterns and the raising of the vocal pitch. . . ."

Prognosis is generally considered poor. However, it is dependent upon the stage to which the virilizing of the folds has progressed, the age of the patient, and her capacity (control of the voice) to restore this disturbed functioning with the needed compensatory actions. It has been thought (Damsté, 1964) that in women under fifty-five years of age a somewhat satisfactory result can be obtained.

Laryngopathia Gravidarum

This is the name given by Kecht (1951) to a voice disturbance that may occur in pregnancy. At this time a light edema of the vocal folds may occur due to the effect of a larger production of estrogen. This vocal disturbance is similar to the type of hoarseness noted in women during the premenstrual period, but the voice quality in laryngopathia gravidarum is lower in pitch and rougher and can be very serious. There may be a strong swelling of the epithelium of the ventricle folds and the aryepiglottic folds, sometimes with hemorrhages and loosening or abrasion of the epithelium. The effect of such a disorder can be complete aphonia, stridor, and dyspnea. However, after deliverance the disturbed areas usually return to their normal healthy states.

Hypothyroidism (Retarded Function of the Thyroid)

Such a disorder may lead to dwarfism and mental retardation (cretinism) when it occurs at a very young age. At a later age it causes myxedema, a thickening of the subcutaneous tissue (Luchsinger and Arnold, 1965). In hypothyroidism the voice is monotonous, low, dull, and has a small range. Speech is slow and articulation is poor. Laryngeal growth has been limited, and the larynx is infantile in development. There is also some suggestion that hypotonia is present and degenerative change of the muscle tissue of the vocal folds has occurred.

Hyperthyroidism

Although symptomotology varies a great deal, there is a tendency for the voice to be of high pitch. However, it is rather unstable and is quickly fatigued. Because of the fast rate of speech and the poor coordination between the respiratory and glottis muscles, the individual with this disorder may develop hoarseness after a great deal of talking. The symptoms have a clear connection with the toxicity of the hormone which causes irritability and tension in the patient (Luchsinger and Arnold, 1965).

Chronic Adrenocortical Insufficiency (Addison's Disease)

The muscular weakness which is typical of this disorder manifests itself in the voice. The initial symptoms are severe breathiness and rapid fatigueability. In more progressed cases the patient is aphonic, although he may be able to whisper short phrases. Generally, his respiratory capacity is small.

It would appear evident that malfunction of the endocrine system can have a direct effect on vocal quality. The most outstanding disorders of voice related to an endocrinological etiology are hypogonadism and virilization of the voice in women; although the occurrence of these is infrequent, it nonetheless is a reminder that when one is faced with a voice disturbance the possibility of a hormonal disorder should be an etiological consideration. The case history and laryngoscopic, endocrinological, and radiological examinations should provide the necessary information as to whether or not the initial treatment belongs in the realm of the endocrinologist.

OTHER ORGANIC DEFECTS AND TRAUMA OF THE LARYNX

Organic anomalies or defects of the laryngeal mechanism are seldom the primary cause of a voice disturbance. Generally, the greatest number of voice disorders are functional in nature although there may be some with secondary organic changes. Since some of these disorders are rare and not all are amenable to voice therapy, only a few of these problems will be reviewed in this chapter.

Congenital Defects of the Larynx

Several congenital malformations of the larynx have been described in the literature (Luchsinger and Arnold, 1965). Some of these are congenital asymmetry, laryngeal webbing of the anterior commissure, and hypoplasia of the vocal folds. In addition, laxity of the vocal ligaments should be mentioned. This particular disorder has been noted in young children, particularly girls who exhibit (1) an abnormally low, soft voice, and (2) hyperextensibility of the joints of the fingers, wrists, and elbows.

The diagnosis of congenital defects is based on: (1) the case history, indicating that the vocal quality has been abnormal since very early childhood; (2) the examination of voice function, when there is clear evidence that there are organic limitations; and (3) an examination with a laryngeal mirror showing an abnormality, with confirmation in the X-ray tomogram or laryngogram.

Congenital Asymmetry

This may consist of (1) an unequal size of both vocal folds, (2) an unequal mobility, which can also be explained as a congenital paresis, (3) a difference in the level of the vocal folds, which may be the consequence of the first two factors. Because of the many variables affecting the stiffness, mass, length, and vibratory pattern of the vocal folds, one cannot readily predict the voice quality that may exist in an individual with congenital asymmetry of the laryngeal structure.

This particular congenital anomaly, as a rule, cannot be improved by surgical intervention. The idea of the implantation or injection of a plastic material (Teflon paste) in order to bring the vocal folds to the same level is a consideration. However, there is little experience to date in the use of such synthetic materials with these disorders. Generally, voice therapy would be suggested in order to obtain the best possible functional result with respect to the organic limitations.

Laryngeal Webbing

Laryngeal webs are basically membranous tissues stretched across the anterior portion of the vocal folds which impede the free vibration of the folds. When this disorder is present, the child will have difficulty in phonating, but may also present a more basic disturbance in the respiratory function. Although congenital in most instances, the disorder can also occur because of trauma to the folds, e.g. surgical trauma. Phonation in the congenital cases is usually breathy, lacking chest resonance, too high a pitch, and limited in volume.

The prime therapy for congenital webbing is surgical intervention. Extirpation of the web occurs in two phases. After one side has been cut loose there is a two-week waiting period before removal of the excess tissue from the other cord in order to prevent the wound surfaces from growing together. This procedure often yields disappointing results. A more reliable method, but one which may cause a great deal more discomfort for the patient, is the insertion of a synthetic material between the folds. This has been referred to as the McNaught procedure (1950). Utilizing this method, after the removal of the excess connective tissue in the anterior commissure, a tantalum keel is inserted between the folds and attached with a suture perforating the thyroid cartilage. It is left in place four to six weeks until epithelization in the anterior commissure is complete and there will be no more connective tissue retraction. Because of the complications of the surgical procedures, there is some feeling that surgery is not advisable in cases with minor voice problems and little effect on respiration (Luchsinger and Arnold, 1965).

Other Organic Defects

ATROPHY OF OLD AGE. In the male this can lead to a high falsetto voice. The explanation of this is diminution of the muscle mass of the folds and the increased rigidity of the coni elastici, the vocal ligaments, so that these no longer have the properties necessary for the production of chest register. There are large individual differences in the degree and the age at which this phenomenon appears. It is certainly not a general phenomenon of old age.

CYSTS OF THE VOCAL FOLD. The only cysts of interest to the voice pathologist are the mucous retention cysts and the epithelial cysts, both of which can be side-effects of laryngitis. Their effect on voice function depends upon their localization. Small cysts near the medial rim of the vocal folds may cause diplophonia (a double tone or interrupted tone) because the vibrating masses on both sides of the glottis are not equal. Opening and removal of the wall of the cysts is done with micro-laryngeal surgery in order to save the connective tissue and muscular layers. After surgery, as a rule, a period of voice therapy is necessary in order to modify vocal habits which have formed during the existence of the cysts.

PROLAPS OF THE VENTRICLE. This disorder is hyperplasia of the mucous membrane which may cover a part of the vocal fold. The most likely cause is chronic coughing and pressing. Therapy consists in cauterization or extirpation of the excessive tissues, mucous membrane, and possibly reeducation of vocal habits which have led to the coughing and pressing.

LARYNGOCELE. This is an enlargement of the lumen of the ventricle which may bulge in lateral and cranial directions. It is of rare occurrence, sometimes being seen in glass blowers and patients with carcinoma of the vocal folds, probably because for many years they have had the habit of speaking and coughing with a high subglottic pressure.

TUBERCULOSIS AND SYPHILIS OF THE LARYNX. These specific inflammations of the larynx have become so rare that they are hardly seen in practice. This, however, may increase the risk of not recognizing them, so that in each case of doubt an Xray examination of the chest and appropriate blood tests should be performed.

GRANULOMA. This is a tumor-like mass of granulation tissue which arises as a reaction to repeated damage of the epithelium of the posterior commissure. It is sometimes seen following intubation narcosis. Trauma, by misuse of the voice, is probably a supporting factor. It has been noted that a granuloma may disappear under strict vocal rest.

PAPILLOMATOSIS OF THE LARYNX. In children, multiple papillomas (small wart-like growths) occur on the vocal folds, with possible extension over the epiglottis, the ventricular folds, and the trachea. A virus is suspected as a possible etiological factor. There is a strong tendency for the epithelial tumors to recur even after removal. An assumption is that continuous microtrauma, by misuse of the voice, may be a growth stimulant for the papillomata.

The laryngoscopic diagnosis of papillomatosis is further enhanced by a histological examination of a biopsy. The prognosis becomes more favorable with advancing age. Usually on reaching adulthood, changes for recurrence and spreading are greatly reduced. At that time, however, the many surgical interventions may have caused a lasting situation of cicatrization and stenosis. Because of this, the therapeutic methodologies employed should be as conservative as possible, particularly in children. Surgery for removal of the papillomata should be considered only when urgent conditions, such as stridor or imminent dyspnea, occur and then with great care that layers under the epithelium will not be damaged. Cryotherapy has been an important improvement in the surgical removal of papillomata because it is a fairly conservative surgical approach in that it does not cause extensive scarring or damage. The freezing, by liquid nitrogen, of the subepithelial layer is followed by revulsion or involution of the papilloma. Following surgical intervention, voice therapy is indicated to teach the child to use his voice as effectively as possible in order to prevent any further traumatization.

The adult type of papilloma is usually solitary (occurring on one place only) and has no tendency to recur after it has been removed. The usual location is the anterior half of one vocal fold. Therapy consists of removal by direct laryngoscopy. The removed tissue has to be histologically examined in order to exclude malignancy.

TRAUMA OF THE LARYNX. The larynx is rather well-protected against external force. However, due to the increasing number of traffic accidents, the frequency of laryngeal trauma has increased. In such cases (where the laryngeal area is traumatized by a strong blow from or against some object, such as a dashboard or motorcycle handlebars) cartilagenous fractures, torn ligaments or a ruptured trachea may occur. The immediate consequences are usually haematoma in the neck and swellings of the larynx. This may eventually lead to luxation (dislocation), with hemarthrosis of the cricoarytenoid joint and emphysema of the neck, which may extend to the face and thorax. There may exist a condition of vital danger in which tracheotomy is indicated. Trauma to the larynx could also be due to surgical intervention, e.g. emergency tracheotomy. Any trauma to the larynx resulting in mucous membrane adhesions, dislocation in the cricothyroid or cricoarytenoid joints may have very damaging effects on the larynx, limiting the vibrational patterns of the folds and causing a loss of control of the vocal folds, such as tension factors. Such structural deviations and limitations will almost definitely result in phonatory disorders.

In children the effect of high tracheotomy may sometimes damage the cricoid cartilage. The consequence of such damage if not prevented is usually subglottic stenosis with irrepairable damage to the respiratory function and phonation. The child must then wear a cannula and the damage to the cricoid cartilage results in a structural deviation. With the development of a stenosis, efforts at decannulation become difficult in certain cases, if at all possible.

Children who wear a cannula because of laryngeal stenosis do not learn to phonate in the normal manner. They usually develop a "Donald Duck" type of speech. Because of the involvement of the tongue in this type of speech pattern, articulation is greatly limited, and these children are usually intelligible only to those individuals having very frequent contact with them.

A really functional surgery of the larynx, directed towards the restoration of physiological relations, does not yet exist. It is possible, however, to reconstruct a lumen in an obstructed larynx, but this is not a simple matter (Bennett, 1960). Reconstruction must be concerned with respiration, phonation, and swallowing. From a strictly phonatory point of view, certain minimum conditions must be present. In other words, there must be an open connection between the trachea and the hypopharynx, and artificial (created by surgery) vocal folds must be present. The surgeon may try to improve the conditions for phonation by implanting a piece of cartilage or injection of Teflon suspension in these folds in order to bring them more toward the median. Some clinical experience has suggested that if an individual can succeed in vibrating such a fold by the breath stream, the continued use of this mechanism will make phonation easier. It is felt that phonation itself adapts the form of the fold to its function. The assumption is that this can be ascribed to the Bernoulli effect, where the constant suction force of the air stream aids in building up a broad vocal fold from the narrow one created surgically.

Such instances are indeed rare, but when they occur it is of utmost importance that voice therapy and reeducation in the use of the voice be instituted as soon as possible.

Chapter 8

CARCINOMA OF THE LARYNX

APPROXIMATELY 2500 TO 4000 people undergo surgical removal of the larynx (laryngectomy) each year. The primary etiological factor for such a drastic step is cancer of the larynx. The disease is more common among people of middle age (fifty years) and over, and occurs mostly in men. "Reports on sex ratio have varied from as many as nine to fourteen males to every one female . . ." (Lerman, 1972). Since the mortality rate due to cancer of the larynx is very low, prognosis for this disease is better than for many other forms of carcinoma. Although the etiology of cancer of the larynx is still unknown several factors have been suggested: genetic factors; chronic irritation, as caused by air pollution and by excessive use of tobacco and alcohol; and certain forms of chronic hyperplastic laryngitis may develop into carcinoma. Although rare, physical trauma to the larynx may also necessitate a laryngectomy.

The first symptoms of carcinoma of the larynx is hoarseness. But, since hoarseness is such a common symptom occurring in so many conditions that affect the vocal folds, it can function to conceal carcinoma as well as reveal it. Therefore, vocal fold cancer may remain unnoticed for a long period of time in spite of this early overt symptom. In cases where individuals make excessive use of tobacco or alcohol there may already exist a cough (smoker's cough) or hoarseness, together with an excess of mucous. Under these circumstances the hoarseness must become very severe before the individual sees reason to consult a physician. It should, therefore, be looked upon also as a "rule" that when hoarseness persists for a period of six weeks or more, the patient should immediately be referred to a laryngologist for a thorough laryngoscopic examination.

DIAGNOSIS

When viewing via indirect laryngoscopy, the deviation seen in the larynx may vary from a slight local discoloration and thickening of one vocal fold to a cauliflower-like or ulcerous tumor which covers both halves of the larynx, narrows the lumen, and extends above and below the glottis. It has proven useful, in terms of prognostic indications and treatment, to describe the deviation in terms of: localization (supraglottic, glottic, sub-glottic) and form (papillomatous, infiltrative, ulcerous), and spreading (stages I through IV) (Struben, 1961). The final diagnosis is based on the case history and laryngoscopy and biopsy findings, the latter enabling us to differentiate between malignant growths and benign tumors.

As previously stated, the prognosis of carcinoma of the larynx is generally quite favorable. There is a tendency for the tumor not to disseminate (except in the very advanced stages), and in more than half the cases (all factors such as age, early diagnosis versus late diagnosis, present health of the patient included), therapeutic procedures are very successful.

MEDICAL TREATMENT

Radiotherapy with high voltage Xray or radioactive Cobalt has had fairly good results in cancers which are limited to one vocal fold, as long as that fold is not fixated. Stroboscopic laryngoscopy has been utilized in checking the results of radiation therapy. If normal vibrations of the vocal fold do not reappear, it is doubtful that the tumor has been completely eradicated.

Narrow field surgery, laryngofissure, and hemi-laryngectomy, although still performed, occur less frequently than in the past. A possible reason for this is that as soon as the growth has infiltrated so far as to have exceeded the limits of radiotherapy, it is usually necessary to perform more extensive surgery. Sometimes partial laryngectomy is attempted with the risk of subsequent deglutition accidents. In a complete or total laryngectomy, the entire larynx (all the cartilages, their connections, and intrinsic musculature) is removed. The hyoid bone may or may not be included. Pressman (Snidecor, 1962) also states that "the attached extrinsic muscles coming from the sternum to the larynx and from the larynx to the hyoid bone are usually included" in a total laryngectomy. Because such a procedure removes one of the organs associated with respiration, a tracheostoma must be created in the neck to allow for respiration.

The total laryngectomy has far-reaching anatomical physiological consequences for the patient: (1) Because of the removal of all the necessary structures for normal speech, normal voice and even whispering are not possible; (2) the (normal) secretions once expelled through the pharyngeal and oral cavities are now brought up through the tracheostoma; (3) breathing will be slightly altered, in that air is now inspired and expired through the tracheostoma; (4) while bathing or showering the individual has to take special precautions in order to prevent the intrusion of water in the trachea, and; (5) other changes affecting smell, taste, smoking, etc. will occur. As one patient so astutely stated, "My nose is on my neck."

Immediately after the operation the patient is left with no voice. He makes attempts, but finds that although his mouth seems to move, no speech sounds are forthcoming. However, the laryngectomized individual can learn to speak again by using esophageal speech and/or an artificial larynx. Other methods have been referred to, e.g. buccal and pharyngeal speech, but these are not prefered, as they tend to distort speech and render it less intelligible. More recently, however, two methods have been devised in an attempt to eliminate the learning of esophageal speech and the use of the artificial larynx.

One of these has been developed by Asai of Japan and has has commonly been referred to as the *Asai Technique*. The surgical technique consists of three stages or operations following

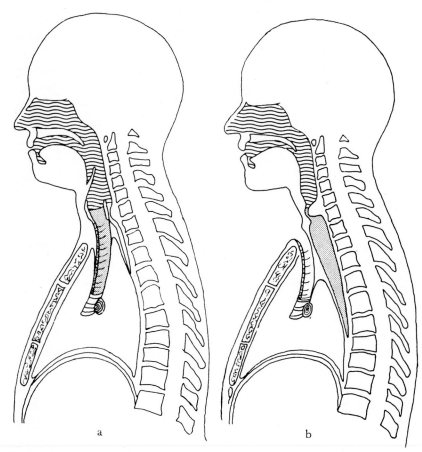

Figure 8. Anatomical situation before and after laryngectomy. After laryngectomy the food- and airways are separated completely. The esophagus takes over the bellows function of the lungs for the purpose of speaking.

the removal of the larynx. Very basically, the procedure involves constructing a tube (dermal) extending from the upper portion of the trachea to the hypopharynx. Air can then be expired through this tube, placing the pseudoglottis into vibration. Various clinical reports have indicated that the voice quality obtained with this procedure is superior to that of esophageal speech. There are, however, certain disadvantages to this technique. First, one is

required to have three more operations following the laryngectomy, with the resultant convalescent period and added financial
burden. Second, in order for the patient to talk, he must use
his hand to close off the tracheal opening. The third disadvantage,
pointed out by Miller (1969), is that the patient "has to
manually press the skin over the upper end of the dermal tube,
sometimes when swallowing saliva or liquid foods." Some patients
have reported reactions from slight annoyance to being repulsed
by this. Currently the Asai operation has not reached the great
proportions predicted for it earlier. This may be because the
technique is not yet widespread among surgeons and/or it has
not been proven to be any more successful than a total laryngectomy alone.

More recently Taub (1970) has devised a prosthetic larynx.
This new larynx is U-shaped and it "contains a varying-frequency
flapper type feed for phonation, and a one-way air valve. The
ultimate plan for fitting is to attach it at one end by a tube to
the tracheostomy and at the other end to a fistula running from
the anterolateral neck to the hypopharynx. The fistula will be
created by a standard esophagostomy." It is felt that with such a
device the laryngectomized individual will be able to produce
a more normal sounding voice with very little training.

Certain problems may be encountered utilizing this prosthetic
larynx. First, it requires a second operative procedure for those
laryngectomees who have not developed a postoperative fistula.
Although the procedure itself is a minor one, certain factors such
as the ability of the tissues to support the procedure and the
reoccurrence of carcinoma must first be considered. It would
also appear that each patient would require an individual fitting
of the device and that this may require an extensive period of
time.

SPEECH REHABILITATION

The most vivid aspect of a total laryngectomy is that the
patient can no longer produce normal voice. Initially the patient
makes attempts to produce normal voice, which usually leads to

undesirable form of speech called the "pseudowhisper." It is important that the patient receive therapy as soon as is medically advisable.

The Artificial Larynx

The first patient who underwent a successful laryngectomy (by Billroth in 1873) was fitted with an artificial larynx designed by Billroth's assistant, Gussenbauer. It was of the pneumatic type. In the pneumatic or reed type of artificial larynx, one end of a tube is placed in or on the trachestoma, which channels air from the stoma to the other end of the pipe which is held in the mouth. In its travel the air passes over a reed, producing the vibrations necessary for speech. (Taub's prosthetic larynx is basically a pneumatic larynx.) Although this type of larynx is still in use today (Lauder, 1969), it has been generally replaced by the electronic larynx.

In the electronic or electro-larynx the sound vibrations are set up in the pharyngeal and oral cavities by placing the head of the instrument against the skin of the neck or directly under the jaw. The device itself is a vibrator powered by batteries. The head of the instrument is basically a diaphragm which imparts sharp sound impulses which are transmitted into the oral and pharyngeal cavities.

There are both advantages and disadvantages to the electro-larynx. Most individuals can learn to speak with this type of artificial larynx within a few hours of training, and this enables them to have almost immediate communicative ability. The sound of the apparatus, however, is mechanical and monotonous. Although studies concerning intelligibility and preference of artificial larynx versus esophageal speech have not been con- clusive, there is some feeling that the noise generated by the artificial larynx distorts voiceless consonants and may mask the speech produced (Hyman, 1955; McCroskey and Mulligan, 1963; Snidecor, 1962: 152; Shames, et al. 1962). In addition, the use of the device tends to draw unwanted attention to the apparatus and the person.

Another dispute which exists relates to when the artificial

larynx should be introduced (Shanks, 1971). Some authorities suggest that the artificial larynx is advocated only for those patients who have been unable to learn esophageal speech. Diedrich (1966) in particular advocates the use of the artificial larynx the first time the patient starts to receive therapy, the contention being that it gives the patient immediate communication, and prepares him, via phrasing and articulation, for learning esophageal speech.

Esophageal Speech

The method of speaking preferred for the laryngectomized patient is esophageal speech. Diedrich and Youngstrom (1965) define it as follows: "Esophageal speech is that in which the vicarious air chamber is located within the lumen of the esophagus and the neoglottis is located above (cephalad) the air chamber. The site of the neoglottis is the pharyngo-esophageal segment or junction and may contain fibers of the inferior constrictor, cricopharyngeus, and/or the superior esophageal sphincter which are predominantly located at C5 and C6." Most authorities (Damsté, 1958; Snidecor, 1962; Robe, et al. 1956a, 1956b) are in agreement as to the site of neoglottis, except for the work presented by Micheli-Pelligrini (1957).

In esophageal speech, air is first pumped down into the esophagus. It is then returned and on passing the folds of the esophageal sphincter is brought into vibration. The dynamics of air intake have been studied and viewed in many cineflorographic studies, Damsté (1958) and Diedrich and Youngstrom (1966) being only two. However, the expulsion of air is still not completely known.

Moolenaar-Bijl (1953a, 1953b) discovered that the plosive consonants (p,t,k) play an important role in the production of esophageal speech. The utilization of these consonants, and more recently the (s) consonant, to facilitate the production of esophageal speech have been referred to as the "Injection" or "PTK" method. It is based on the fact that air in the esophagus is replenished by the articulation pressure of these consonants

(Van den Berg, et al., 1956). Damsté (1958) feels that the technique can be taught to the patients in the following steps:

1. After a simple anatomical explanation, with the help of a rough sketch, the patient is asked if he can belch or burp. In the past the use of such terminology (burp or belch) drew negative comments from speech clinicians; however, if the patient has some point of reference as to what esophageal speech sounds like, this may make teaching the initial sound much more simple. It is explained to the patient that this is the basis, the foundation for his new way of speaking.
2. Assuming the patient has difficulty, he is then taught how he can displace minute quantities of air by movements of the tongue, etc. then there should be no difficulty in producing a clearly explosive /p/.
3. The patient is asked to articulate the stop-consonants (p,t,k). In other words, the patient is asked to build up some pressure in the oral-pharyngeal area before production of these consonants. If this is done correctly, air is constantly injected into the esophagus and sooner or later an esophageal sound will be produced. Then monosyllabic words containing the plosive sounds are practiced .

These three steps represent one therapeutic methodology in establishing the basic esophageal sound. Diedrich (1971) presents another approach utilizing the plosive sounds. Therapy must not end here, although in the past clinicians have been satisfied with teaching the laryngectomee the basic sound, some monosyllabic words, and then dismissing them from therapy. Therapy must continue through monosyllabic words to polysyllabic ones: phrases, sentences, improved articulation, phrasing, inflection, pitch, and loudness (Rigrodsky, et al., 1971).

The length of time it takes the laryngectomee to learn esophageal speech varies, but with all factors being favorable, it is possible to learn to produce the esophageal sound within the first two training sessions. Within one to three months he should be able to use esophageal speech successfully outside the clinical situation and for communication purposes. With continued therapy and practice, more improvement may be noted.

DIFFICULTIES EXPERIENCED IN ACQUISITION
OF ESOPHAGEAL SPEECH

Studies have indicated that many laryngectomees do not learn esophageal speech. The reasons may be physical, psychological, or in some instances, the clinician's inability to deal with the difficulties that may arise in teaching the laryngectomee.

One of the most common problems is the inability of the laryngectomee to relax the sphincter of the esophagus at the moment that the air has to pass in one direction or in another. One can detect this by watching the laryngectomee "snapping" at the air and trying to push it back. The air usually does not proceed any further than the pharynx. On other occasions the air can be heard entering the esophagus, but the attempt to produce sound by the patient is in vain, and the air usually passes on through the esophagus to enter the stomach. If this occurs often enough, the patient usually has a very uncomfortable feeling. In such instances relaxation exercises may aid in reducing the amount of pharyngeal constriction, thereby enabling production of the esophageal sound. In cases of greater difficulty, some physicians have gone so far as to insert a catheter to insufflate the esophagus in hopes of overcoming the reflex contraction of the sphincter. However, this is not generally advisable.

Research is still not definite concerning the relationship between the type of surgical procedure utilized and the quality of the esophageal voice. Regardless of the perfection of techniques by the laryngectomee, he is still dependent upon the postsurgical results (scar tissue and its mucosal lining). Lateral X-rays of the neck made during phonation with esophageal voice, after swallowing a contrast material, show the contours of a contracting cricopharyngeaus muscle and the sphincter of the esophagus (Damsté, 1958). At that point where the canal narrows into the pharynx, the sound is generated by successive releases of air bubbles and the clapping together of the epithelium walls and its covering mucus. If a diverticulum (sac or pouch) of the pharyngeal wall is present, this may tend to collect mucous, which in turn influences the esophageal sound by giving it a "moist" and "bubbling" character. A diverticulum cannot always be prevented even if the pharyngeal wall has been sutured with the greatest care. Leakage of saliva may produce a small fistula which later heals in the form of a diverticulum.

In some speakers an audible sound (blowing noise) from the tracheostoma has a masking effect on the esophageal speech of the individual. This may be caused by (1) uncontrolled expulsion of breath in patients using poor techniques of speaking; (2) anatomically unfavorable conditions of the P-E (pharyngo-esophageal) junction, which causes patients to put more effort into the production of esophageal voice; and (3) a presbyacusic type of hearing loss in older patients which makes it less likely that they will hear, and therefore control, the stoma noise. Very clearly, this superfluous noise must be eliminated or reduced in the therapeutic process.

Psychological factors are of great importance in the learning of esophageal speech (Gardner, 1966; Shames, et al., 1963; Lauder, 1969; Levin, 1962). The patient has just been faced with a life and death situation. He has been mutilated and left not as before. His inability to communicate is only one of many fears and anxieties (Stoll, 1958). The speech clinician, with the help of referral sources—the psychologist and social worker in particular—must be able to cope with these feelings if success in therapy is to be attained. The morale and motivation of the laryngectomee is a most important factor in successful speech rehabilitation.

BIBLIOGRAPHY

Alexander, F. M.: *The Use of the Self*. Manchester, Manchester Press, 1955.

Ardran, G. M., and Kemp, F. H.: Closure and opening of the larynx during swallowing. *Br J Radiol, 9*:205-210, 1956.

Ardran, G. M., and Kemp, F. M.: The mechanism of the larynx. Part I: The movements of the arytenoid and cricoid cartilages. *Br J Radiol, 39*:641-654, 1966.

Ardran, G. M., and Kemp, F. H.: Laryngeal function following lateral fixation of a vocal cord. *Br J Disord Commun, 2*:15-22, 1967.

Arnold, G. E.: Vocal nodules and polyps: Laryngeal tissue reaction to habitual hyperkinetic dysphonia. *J Speech Hear Dis, 26*:296-317, 1962.

Arnold, G. E.: Further experiences with intrachordal teflon injection. *Laryngoscope, 74*:802-815, 1964.

Arnold, G. E., and Pinto, S.: Ventricular dysphonia: New interpretation of an old observation. *Laryngoscope, 70*:1608-1627, 1960.

Aronson, A. E.; Brown, J. R.; Litin, E. M., and Pearson, J. S.: Spastic dysphonia. I. Voice, neurologic and psychiatric aspects. *J Speech Hear Dis, 33*:203-218, 1968a.

Aronson, A. E.; Brown, J. R.; Litin, E. M., and Pearson, J. S.: Spastic dysphonia. II. Comparison with essential (voice) tremor and other neurologic and psychogenic dysphonias. *J Speech Hear Dis, 33*:219-231, 1968b.

Ash, J. E.: Pathologic and epithelial changes and tumors of the larynx. In N. M. Levin (Ed.): *Voice and Speech Disorders: Medical Aspects*. Springfield, Thomas, 1962, pp. 66.

Baker, D. C.: Contact ulcer of the larynx. *Laryngoscope, 64*:73-78, 1954.

Bauer, H.: Die dieziehungen der phoniatrie zur endokrinologie. *Folia Phoniatr (Basel), 20*:387-393, 1968.

Baynes, R. A.: An incidence study of chronic hoarseness among children. *J Speech Hear Dis, 31*:172-176, 1966.

Bennett, T.: Laryngeal trauma. *Laryngoscope, 70*:973-982, 1960.

Berendes, J.: Die verantwortlichkeit des arztes bei der anwendung anaboler steriode in hinblick auf die stimme. *Folia Phoniatr (Basel), 20*:379-386, 1968.

Berry, M. F., and Eisenson, J.: *Speech Disorders*. New York, Appleton, 1956.

Bloch, P.: Neuro-psychiatric aspects of spastic dysphonia. *Folia Phoniatr (Basel)*, *17*:301-364, 1965.

Boone, D.: *The Voice and Voice Therapy.* Englewood Cliffs, P-H, 1971.

Bosma, J. F.: Deglutition: Pharyngeal state. *Physiol Rev, 37*:275, 1957.

Bosma, J. F.; Sheets, B.. and Shelton, R.: Tongue, hyoid and larynx displacement in swallowing and phonation. *J Appl Physiol, 15*:283, 1960.

Brewer, D. W.; Briess, F. B., and Faaborg-Andersen, K.: Phonation: Clinical testing versus electromyography. *Ann Otol Rhinol Laryngol, 69*:781, 1960.

Brodnitz. F. S., and Froeschels, E.: Treatment of nodules of vocal cords *J Speech Hear Dis, 23*:112-117, 1958.

Brodnitz, F. S.: Contact ulcer of the larynx. *Arch Otolaryngol, 74*:70, 1961.

Brodnitz, F. S.: *Vocal Rehabilitation*, 3rd ed. Rochester, The American Academy of Opthamology and Otolaryngology, 1965.

Brodnitz, F. S., and Froeschels, D.: Treatment of nodules of vocal cords by the chewing method. *Arch Otolaryngol, 59*:560-565, 1954.

Buch, N. H.: Stroboscopy of the larynx. In *System for Stroboscopic Motion Analysis of the Larynx.* B and K Instruments, Inc., 1972, pp. 3-9.

Buchtal, F., and Faaborg-Andersen, K.: Electromyography of laryngeal and respiratory muscles: Correlation with phonation and respiration. *Ann Otol Rhinol Laryngol, 73*:119, 1964.

Chew, W.: Importance of early diagnosis of hoarseness and its management. *EENT Digest, 28*:63-69, 1966.

Cleary, J. A.: On the ary-epiglottic folds. *Ann Otol Rhinol Laryngol, 63*:960-979, 1954.

Clerf, L. H.: Unilateral vocal cord paralysis. *JAMA*, 1953.

Coleman, R. F.: Decay characteristics of vocal fry. *Folia Phoniatr (Basel), 15*:256-263, 1963.

Coleman, R. F., and Wendahl, R. W.: Vocal roughness and stimulus duration. *Speech Monogr, 34*:85-92, 1967.

Cooker, H. S.: An introduction to sound and the speech and hearing mechanisms. In Weston, A. J. (Ed.): *Communicative Disorders: An Appraisal.* Springfield, Thomas, 1972, pp. 417.

Cornut, G.: Contribution a l'étude clinique et acoustique des dysphonies spastiques. *J Fr Otorhinolaryngol, 14*:439-445, 1965.

Curry, E. T.: Hoarseness and voice changes in male adolescents. *J Speech Hear Dis, 14*:23-25, 1949.

Damsté, P. H.: Esophageal Speech. Thesis, Groningen, Gebr: Hoitsema, 1958.

Damsté, P. H.: Virile changes in the voice by androgens. Boerhaave postgraduate course on side effects of drugs. University of Leiden, Netherlands, 1964a.

Damsté, P. H.: Virilization of the voice due to anabolic stereoids. *Folia Phoniatr (Basel), 16*:10-18, 1964b.

Damsté, P. H.: Voice change in adult women caused by virilizing agents. *J Speech Hear Dis, 32*:126-132, 1967.

Damsté, P. H.: X-ray study of phonation. *Folia Phoniatr (Basel), 20*:64-88, 1968.

Damsté, P. H.; Hollien, H.; Moore, P., and Murry, T.: An x-ray study of vocal fold length. *Folia Phoniatr (Basel), 20*:349-359, 1968.

Darley, F.: *Diagnosis and Appraisal of Communication Disorders.* Englewood Cliffs, P-H, 1964.

Diedrich, W. D.: Primary stage of teaching alaryngeal speech. In Rigrodsky, S., and Lerman, J. (Eds.): *Therapy for the Laryngectomized Patient: A Speech Clinician's Manual.* New York, Tchrs Coll, 1971, pp. 66.

Diedrich, W. D., and Youngstrom, D. A.: *Alaryngeal Speech.* Springfield, Thomas, 1966, pp. 215.

Dedo, H. H., and Dunker, E.: Husson's theory: An experimental analysis of his research data and conclusions. *Arch Otolaryngol, 85*:303, 1967.

Eisenson, J.; Auer, J. J., and Irwin, J. V.: *The Psychology of Communication.* New York, Appleton, 1963.

Faaborg-Andersen, K.: Electromyographic investigation of intrinsic laryngeal muscles in humans. *Acta Physiol Scand (Suppl 140)*, 1957.

Faaborg-Andersen, K.: The position of paretic vocal cords. *Acta Otolaryngol, 57*:50-54, 1964.

Faaborg-Andersen, K., and Sonninen, A.: The function of the extrinsic laryngeal muscles at different pitch. *Acta Otolaryngol, 51*:89-93, 1959.

Faaborg-Andersen, K., and Vennard, W.: Electromyography of extrinsic laryngeal muscles during phonation of different vowels. *Ann Otol Rhinol Laryngol, 73*:248, 1964.

Fairbanks, G.: *Voice and Articulation Drillbook.* New York, Har-Row, 1960.

Fleisch, A.: Die pneumotachographie. In (Ed.): *Handbuch der Biologischen Arbeitsmethoden.* Vienna, Urban and Schwarzenberg, 1933, Vol. III, pp.

Fry, D. B.: Prosodic phenomena. In B. Malmberg (Ed.): *Manual of Phonetics.* Amsterdam, North Holland Pub Co, 1968, pp. 568.

Gardner, W. H.: The whistle technique in esophageal speech. *J Speech Hear Dis, 27*:187-188, 1962.

Gardner, W. H.: Adjustment problems of laryngectomized women. *Arch Otolaryngol, 83*:31-42, 1966.

Gray, C. W., and Wise, C. M.: *The Bases of Speech,* 3rd ed. New York, Har-Row, 1959.

Greene, M.: *The Voice and Its Disorders.* London, Pitman Medical Publ Co, Inc., 1964.

Hanley, M., and Thurman. W. L.: *Developing Vocal Skills.* New York, HRW, 1963.

Heaver, L.: Psychiatric observation of the personality structure of patients with habitual dysphonia. *Logos, 1*:21, 1958.

Hollien, H.: Vocal fold thickness and fundamental frequency of phonation. *J Speech Hear Res, 5*:237-243, 1962a.

Hollien, H.: The relationship of vocal fold length to vocal pitch for female subjects. *Proceedings of the XII International Congress of Logopedics and Phoniatrics.* 1962b, pp. 38-43.

Hollien, H.; Coleman, R., and Moore, P.: Stroboscopic laminography of the larynx. *Acta Otolaryngol, 65*:209-216, 19 .

Hollien, H., and Curtis, J.: Elevation and tilting of vocal folds as a function of vocal pitch. *Folia Phoniatr (Basel), 14*:23-36, 1962.

Hollien, H., and Michel, J. F.: Vocal fry as a phonational register. *J Speech Hear Res, 11*:600-604, 1968.

Hollien, H., and Moore, P.: Measurements of the vocal folds during changes in pitch. *J Speech Hear Res, 3*:157-165, 1960.

Hollien, H.; Moore, P.; Wendahl, R. W., and Michel, J. F.: On the nature of vocal fry. *J Speech Hear Res, 9*:245-247, 1966.

Husson, R.: Etude des phenomenes physiologiques et acoustiques fondamentaux de la voix chantee. Thesis, Paris, 1950.

Husson, R.: *La Voix Chantée.* Paris, Gauthier-Villars, 1960.

Hyman, M.: An experimental study of artificial larynx and esophageal speech. *J Speech Hear Dis, 20*:291-299, 1955.

Jackson, C.: Contact ulcers of the larynx. *Arch Otolaryngol, 22*:1-15, 1935.

Jackson, C.: Contact ulcer of the larynx. *Ann Otolaryngol, 37*:227, 1966.

Jacobson, E.: *You Must Relax.* New York, McGraw, 1934.

Johnson, W.; Darley, F. L., and Spriestersbach, D.: *Diagnostic Methods in Speech Pathology.* New York, Har-Row, 1963.

Judson, L. S. V., and Weaver, A. T.: *Voice Science,* 2nd ed. New York, Appleton, 1965.

Kainz, F.: *De "Sprache" des Tieres.* Stuttgart, F. Enke Verlag, 1961.

Kaplan, H. M.: *Anatomy and Physiology of Speech.* New York, McGraw, 1960.

Kecht, H.: Zur kenntnis der laryngopathia gravidarum. *Laryngol Rhinol Otol, 30*:230, 1951.

Kinsey, A. C.; Pomeroy, W. B., and Martin, G. E.: *Sexual Behavior in the Human Male.* Philadelphia, Saunders, 1948.

Kirchner, F. R.; Toledo, P. S., and Svoboda, D. J.: Studies of the larynx after Teflon injection. *Arch Otolaryngol, 83*:350-354, 1966.

Landman, G. H. M.: Laryngografie en Cinelaryngografie: *De Toepassing van Contrastmiddel in de Rontgendiagnostiek van de Larynx.* Nijmegen, Centrale Drukkerij, 1966a.

Landman, G. H. M.: A roentgencinematographic study of recurrent paralysis. *Pract Otorhinolaryngol (Basel), 29*:294-298, 1966b.

Lauder, E.: *Self-Help for the Laryngectomee*, 2nd ed. 1960, pp. 138.

Lerman, J. W.: Voice disorders. In Weston, A. J. (Ed.): *Communication Disorders: An Appraisal*. Springfield, Thomas, 1972.

Lerman, J. W., and Duffy, R. J.: Recognition of falsetto voice quality. *Folia Phoniatr (Basel)*, 22:21-27, 1970.

Levin, N. M.: *Voice and Speech Disorders: Medical Aspects*. Springfield, Thomas, 1962.

Lorenz, K.: *Ik Sprak met Viervoeters*. Visse, en Vogels. Amsterdam, Ploegsma.

Luchsinger, R.: Falsetto and Vollton der kopfstimme. *Arch Ohr-Nas-Kehlkheilk*, 155:505, 1949.

Luchsinger, R.. and Arnold, G. E.: *Voice, Speech and Language*. Belmont, Wadsworth Pub, 1965.

Martienssen-Lohman, F.: *Der Wis Sende Sanger*. Zurich, Atlantis-Verlag, 1956.

McCrosky, R. L., and Mulligan, M.: The relative intelligibility of esophageal speech and artificial-larynx speech. *J Speech Hear Dis*, 28:37-41, 1963.

McNaught, R. C.: Surgical correction of anterior web of the larynx. *Laryngoscope*, 60:264-272, 1950.

Merkel, C. L.: *Anthropophonik*. Leipzig, 1863.

Michel, J.: Vocal fry and harshness. Doctoral thesis, University of Florida, 1964.

Michel, J.; Hollien, H., and Moore, P.: Speaking fundamental frequency characteristics of 15-, 16-, and 17-year-old girls. *Lang Speech*, 9:46-51, 1966.

Micheli-Pelligrini, V.: On the so-called pseudo-glottis in laryngectomized persons. *J Laryngol*, 71:504, 1957.

Miller, A.: First experiences with the Asai technique for vocal rehabilitation after total laryngectomy. In Snidecor, J. C. (Ed.): *Speech Rehabilitation of the Laryngectomee*, 2nd ed. Springfield, Thomas, 1969, pp. 189.

Moolenaar-Bijl, A.: Connection between consonant articulation and the intake of air in esophageal speech. *Folia Phoniatr (Basel)*, 5:212-225, 1953a.

Moolenaar-Bijl, A.: The importance of certain consonants in esophageal voice after laryngectomy. *Ann Otol Rhinol Laryngol*, 62:679-689, 1953b.

Moore, G. P.: Voice disorders associated with organic abnormalities. In L. E. Travis (Ed.): *Handbook of Speech Pathology*. New York, Appleton, 1957, pp. 653-706.

Moore, G. P.: *Organic Voice Disorders*. Englewood Cliffs, P-H, 1971.

Moore, G. P., and Thompson, C.: Comments on physiology of hoarseness. *Arch Otolaryngol*, 81:97-102, 1965.

Moses, P. J.: *The Voice of Neurosis*. New York, Grune, 1954.

Myerson, M. C.: *The Human Larynx.* Springfield, Thomas, 1964.

Naidr, Von, J.; Zboril, M., and Sevcik, K.: Die Pubertalen veranderungen der stimme bei jungen in verlauf von 5 jahren. *Folia Phoniatr (Basel),* 17:1-18, 1965.

Peacher, G.: Contact ulcer of the larynx. Part III: Etiological factors. *J Speech Dis, 12*:177-178, 1947a.

Peacher, G.: Contact ulcer of the larynx. Part IV: A clinical study of vocal re-education. *J Speech Dis, 12*:179-190, 1947b.

Peroin, A.: Contact ulcer of the larynx. Pathological observations. *Arch Otolaryngol, 17*:741-746, 1933.

Rees, M.: Some variables affecting perceived harshness. *J Speech Hear Res, 1*:155-168, 1958a.

Rees, M.: Harshness and glottal attack. *J Speech Hear Res, 1*:344-349, 1958b.

Rigrodsky, S., and Lerman, J.: *Therapy for the Laryngectomized Patient. A Speech Clinician's Manual.* New York, Tchrs Coll, 1971.

Robe, E.; Brumlik, J., and Moore, P.: A study of spastic dysphonia: Neurological and electroencephalographic abnormalities. *Laryngoscope, 70*:219-245, 1960.

Robe, E. Y.; Moore, P.; Andrews, A. H., Jr., and Holinger, P. H.: A study of the role of certain factors in the development of speech after laryngectomy. I. Type of operation. *Laryngoscope, 66*:173-186, 1956. II. Site of pseudo-glottis. *Laryngoscope, 66*:382-401, 1956.

Rubin, H. J.: The neurochronaxic theory of voice production: A refutation. *Arch Otolaryngol, 71*:913-920, 1960.

Rubin, H. J.: Intracordal injection of silicone in selected dysphonias. *Arch Otolaryngol, 81*:604, 1965a.

Rubin, H. J.: Pitfalls in treatment of dysphonia by intracordal injections of synthetics. *Laryngoscope, 75*:1381, 1965b.

Rubin, H. J.: Treatment of dysphonia due to unilateral recurrent nerve paralysis by the intracordal injection of synthetics. Film, 1966.

Rubin, H. J., and Lehroff, I.: Pathogenesis and treatment of vocal nodules. *J Speech Hear Dis, 27*:150-161, 1962.

Shames, G. H.; Font, J., and Matthews, J.: Factors related to speech proficiency of the laryngectomized. *J Speech Hear Dis, 28*:273-287, 1963.

Shanks, J. C.: The use of the manufactured larynx for alaryngeal speech training. In Rigrodsky, S., and Lerman, J. (Eds.): *Therapy for the Laryngectomized Patients A Speech Clinician's Manual.* New York, Tchrs Coll, 1971, pp. 66.

Snidecor, J. C.: *Speech Rehabilitation of the Laryngectomized.* Springfield, Thomas, 1962.

Sonesson, B.: Die funktionelle anatomie des cricoarytannoid gelenkes. *Z Anat Entwicklungsgesch, 121*:292-303, 1959.

Sonesson, B.: The functional anatomy of the speech organs. In B. Malmberg (Ed.): *Manual of Phonetics.* Amsterdam, North Holland Pub Co, 1968, pp. 568.

Sonninen, A.: The role of the external-laryngeal muscles. Length-adjustments of the vocal cords in singing. *Acta Otolaryngol* [*Suppl* 130] (*Stockh*), 1956.

Sonninen, A.: The significance of "tracheal bending" and "esophageal opening" in high-pitched singing. *Proc 13th International Congress of Logo Phoniatr,* 1965.

Steer, M. D., and Hanley, T. D.: Instruments of diagnosis, therapy, and research. In (Ed.): *Handbook of Speech Pathology.* New York, Appleton, 1957, pp.

Stoll, B.: Psychological factors determining the success or failure of the rehabilitation program of laryngectomized patients. *Ann Otol Rhinol Laryngol,* 67:550-557, 1958.

Struben, W. H.: *Over de Behandeling van het Larynx Carcinoon.* Thesis, U of Amsterdam, 1961.

Taub, S.: New prosthetic larynx. *Roche Medical Image and Commentary,* 1970.

Timcke, R. H.; von Leden, H., and Moore, P.: Laryngeal vibrations: Measurements of the glottic wave, Part I. The normal vibratory cycle. *Arch Otolaryngol,* 68:1-19, 1958.

Timcke, R. H.; von Leden, H., and Moore, P.: Laryngeal vibrations: Measurements of the glottic wave. Part II. Physiologic variations. *Arch Otolaryngol,* 69:438-444, 1959.

Van den Berg, J. W.: Myoelastic-aerodynamic theory of voice production. *J Speech Hear Res,* 1:227-244, 1958.

Van den Berg, J. W.: The larynx and laryngeal vibrations. In B. Malmberg (Ed.): *Manual of Phonetics.* Amsterdam, North Holland Pub Co, 1968, pp. 568.

Van den Berg, J. W.; Damsté, P. H., and Moolenaar-Bijl, A.: Oesophageal Speech (film). Groningen, The Netherlands, 1956.

Van Riper, C.: *Speech Correction: Principles and Methods,* 4th ed. Englewood Cliffs, P-H, 1963.

Van Riper, C., and Irwin, J. V.: *Voice and Articulation.* Englewood Cliffs, P-H, 1958.

Von Leden, H.: Sound production in man: Objective measures of laryngeal function and phonation. *Ann NY Acad Sci,* 155:56-67, 1968.

Von Leden, H.; Yanaghihara, N., and Werner-Kukuk, E.: Teflon in unilateral vocal cord paralysis. *Arch Otolaryngol,* 85:666-674, 1967.

Waar, C. H., and Damsté, P. H.: Het Fonetogram. *Logopedie en Foniatrie* (Groningen), 40:198-201, 1968.

Wendahl, R. W.: Laryngeal analog synthesis of filter and shimmer auditory parameter of harshness. *Folia Phoniatr* (*Basel*), 18:98-108, 1966.

Wendahl, R. W.; Moore, P., and Hollien, H.: Comments on vocal fry. *Folia Phoniatr (Basel)*, *15*:251-255, 1963.

Wilson, K. D.: Children with vocal nodules. *J Speech Hear Dis*, *26*:19-26, 1961.

Wilson, K. D.: Voice reeducation of adolescents with vocal nodules. *Arch Otolaryngol*, *76*:68-73, 1962.

Winckel, F.: Phoniatric acoustics. In Luchsinger, R., and Arnold, G. E. (Eds.): *Voice, Speech and Language*. Belmont, Wadsworth Pub, 1965, pp. 812.

Wood, K. S.: Terminology and nomenclature. In (Ed.): *Handbook of Speech Pathology*. New York, Appleton, 1957, pp.

Yanaghihara, N.: Experimental observations on the noisy quality of hoarseness. *Studia Phonolog*, *3*:46-57, 1964.

Yanaghihara, N.: Hoarseness: Investigation of the physiological mechanisms. *Ann Otolaryngol*, *76*:472-488, 1967a.

Yanaghihara, N.: Significance of harmonic changes and noise components in hoarseness. *J Speech Hear Res*, *10*:531-541, 1967b.

Zemlin, W. R.: *Speech and Hearing Science: Anatomy and Physiology*. Englewod Cliffs, P-H, 1968.

Zenker, W., and Zenker, A.: Uber die regelung der stimmlippenspannung durch von aussen eingreifende mechanismen. *Folia Phoniatr (Basel)*, *12*:1-36, 1960.

Zumsteeg, H.: Larvierte formen von mutationsstorungen. *Vox*, *26*:   , 1916.

INDEX

A

Abduction, 9
Acoustic research, 27
Addison's disease, 83
Adduction, 9
Alexander, 67
Aphonia, 52
Ardran, 7, 12
Arnold, 25, 56, 66, 77, 79, 83, 84, 86
Aronson, 54
Artificial larynx, 95
Aryepiglottic folds, 8, 12
Arytenoid cartilage, 4, 6
Asai, 92
Ash, 56

B

Baker, 60
Bauer, 80
Baynes, 52
Bennett, 89
Berendes, 80
Bernoulli effect, 14
Berry, 23
Bloch, 54
Boone, 61, 66
Bosma, 12
Breath control, 64
Breathiness, 49
Brewer, 35
Brodnitz, 57, 58, 60, 62, 67, 76
Buch, 74
Buchtal, 35
Buess, 35

C

Carcinoma, 90
Cartilages, larynx, 4

Case history, 22
Castration, 79
Chew, 51
Chest register, 16
Chronic laryngitis, 61, 62
Cleary, 8
Clerf, 9
Coleman, 30, 33, 50, 51
Congenital asymmetry, 84
Congenital defects, 84
Contact ulcer, 59
Conus elasticus, 4, 8
Cooker, 16
Corniculates, 4
Cornut, 54
Coughing reflex, 12
Cricoarytenoid joint, 6
Cricoid cartilage, 4, 6
Cricopharyngeus muscle, 11
Cricothyroid joint, 7
Cricothyroid muscle, 4, 10
Cuneiforms, 4
Curry, 40
Curtis, 7, 33
Cysts, 86

D

Damsté, 17, 34, 80, 82, 96, 97, 98
Darley, 22, 23, 24
Dedo, 14
Diagnosis, 26
Diedrich, 96, 97
Digastricus muscle, 10
Duffy, 43
Dunker, 14
Dysphonia, 48

E

Edema, 58

109